MW00465400

BANISH BEDTIME BATTLES

Banish Bedtime Battles

The Ultimate Six-Week Plan to Help Your
School-Aged Child Sleep Independently

Ellen Flannery-Schroeder, PhD,

and Chelsea Tucker, PhD

ROWMAN & LITTLEFIELD
Lanham • Boulder • New York • London

Published by Rowman & Littlefield
An imprint of The Rowman & Littlefield Publishing Group, Inc.
4501 Forbes Boulevard, Suite 200, Lanham, Maryland 20706
www.rowman.com

86-90 Paul Street, London EC2A 4NE

British Library Cataloguing in Publication Information Available

Library of Congress Cataloging-in-Publication Data
Names: Flannery-Schroeder, Ellen, author. | Tucker, Chelsea, author.
Title: Banish bedtime battles : the ultimate six-week plan to help your school-aged child sleep independently / Ellen Flannery-Schroeder, PhD and Chelsea Tucker, PhD.
Description: Lanham : Rowman & Littlefield, [2024] | Includes bibliographical references and index.
Identifiers: LCCN 2023051691 (print) | LCCN 2023051692 (ebook) | ISBN 9781538187890 (cloth) | ISBN 9781538187906 (ebook)
Subjects: LCSH: Bedtime. | Parent and child. | Child development.
Classification: LCC HQ784.B43 F573 2024 (print) | LCC HQ784.B43 (ebook) | DDC 649/.6—dc23/eng/20240213
LC record available at https://lccn.loc.gov/2023051691
LC ebook record available at https://lccn.loc.gov/2023051692

♾️™ The paper used in this publication meets the minimum requirements of American National Standard for Information Sciences—Permanence of Paper for Printed Library Materials, ANSI/NISO Z39.48-1992.

Dedicated to the many families who have entrusted us with the privilege of guiding them toward greater bedtime empowerment, harmony, and rest.

Contents

Authors' Note ix

Introduction 1

Week 1: Everything You Need to Know about Child Sleep. . .7

Week 2: Parenting: What's Your Style? 35

Week 3: Build Your Child's Coping Skills. 55

Week 4: Pick Your Battles 75

Week 5: You're Ready, Set, Go! 99

Week 6: Battle No More. 139

Bonus Week: Now It's Your Turn! 157

Sleep Resources for Parents 173

Notes. 175

Bibliography 181

Index. 187

About the Authors. 195

Authors' Note

Banish Bedtime Battles presents information collected from research data, personal experiences, clinical experiences, and an author-conducted survey. Client privacy and confidentiality are of utmost importance to the authors. All vignettes included are fictional and were developed as composites of a variety of clients and families seen in the authors' professional practices. The survey was conducted anonymously, and participant data is for educational purposes only.

This book is intended to empower parents and their children to take charge of their bedtime. This book should not be considered a substitute for medical or behavioral health care. Consult a licensed healthcare provider about any diagnostic or healthcare concerns. The authors are not responsible for any adverse effects that individuals may allege as a direct or indirect result of information contained within this book.

Please note, for convenience and readability, we use the term "parent" throughout this book to refer to the many types of caregivers who support children at bedtime.

Introduction

You probably picked up this book because you are one of the sleep-deprived parents struggling to get your child to go to sleep independently. You are exhausted, relying on coffee to get you through the day, easily irritated, and falling asleep in seconds flat the moment you cease movement—wherever and whenever that might be. You are tired of disagreements with your partner about how to handle bedtime battles with your child. You miss the evening relaxation, bedroom privacy, and intimacy with your partner you had before kids. It's no wonder that parents of children with sleep disturbance are more likely to experience marital issues, anxiety, and even depression.[1]

Research suggests that most families struggle with bedtime difficulties at one time or another. In September 2022, we conducted a survey of 146 parents of children age four to thirteen and found that 94 percent of parents reported having a child currently experiencing at least one of the six "battle" types addressed in this book. Additionally, we found that although 80 percent of parents reported that their children have established bedtime routines, 86 percent fail to follow the bedtime routine each night. Finally, the survey offers validity to the types of bedtime battles reviewed in this book—with the most common battle type being reported by 65 percent of parents and the least common battle type reported by 46 percent of parents. Thus, substantial numbers of parents and children are struggling with bedtime problems each night.

The good news is that you are not alone, and now is the time to begin to solve your problem. We will walk you through a six-week plan to gradually and painlessly get your child in their bed and you in yours without the bedtime battles. We'll give you full nights of uninterrupted sleep *and* help you feel like a competent, loving parent.

Banish Bedtime Battles stands out among all the sleep and parenting books. No other book like it exists. While there are numerous books written for helping young children get to sleep and even more on parenting topics, this is the one and only book for helping *school-aged* children to sleep independently.

When we talk about *independent sleep*, we want to be clear about what we mean. An independent sleeper is a child who can fall asleep in their designated sleeping location on their own, without the intervention of other people or sleep aids, and remains there throughout the night. The designated sleeping location will differ across homes—in some, children may be sleeping on a couch, others may have their own bed in their own room, still others may share a bed with a sibling. Your child does not need their own bedroom, or even their own bed, to become an independent sleeper. They need only to drift off to sleep on their own in the sleeping space that is intended for them.

You might think that the main benefits of independent sleep are the blissful zzzs that you and your child will get. While that *is* a highly valued outcome, there are other crucial perks that will come out of this six-week journey. Your child will get more and higher quality sleep. Better sleep is associated with better concentration, increased ability to control behavior, and higher academic achievement.[2] Your child will become more self-reliant, competent, and confident. Learning to sleep independently requires children to develop several coping skills necessary for good psychological adjustment and well-being. Your independent sleeper will come to learn that they are capable of navigating situations on their own, using parents as touchstones only when necessary. Your child will be able to use these skills across many situations that will help them successfully navigate their world with confidence and a sense of accomplishment. This six-week plan is for parents who want their child to sleep independently in the child's bed. (*Note*: we will use the word "bed" to refer to where the child sleeps for the remainder of this book.) This six-week plan is for parents of school-aged children whose sleep difficulties are behavioral in nature, driven by nighttime fears, or are simply a result of longtime habits, and who have independent sleep as the goal for their children. This six-week plan *is not* intended to address sleep disorders including narcolepsy, sleep apnea, restless leg syndrome, sleepwalking, sleep terrors, or nightmare disorder; see Week 1 for more information on childhood sleep disorders. This six-week plan *does not* involve "cry it out" methods, punishments, or physical means of establishing nighttime separation (e.g., locking parental bedroom door).

Instead, we present positive psychology methods such as positive reinforcement, promotion of effective parenting behaviors, instruction in child coping strategies, and the establishment of bedtime routines. Helping your child become an independent sleeper involves a focus on changing behaviors—your child's *and* yours.

Banish Bedtime Battles offers specific information about how to (1) engage in effective parenting strategies and (2) train your child to cope with discomfort. These two essential skills are not only a critical part of the solution to bedtime problems, but they are also transferable beyond bedtime hours. When parenting skills are sharpened, child behavior improves and parent-child relationships grow stronger. As you help your child to use the coping skills to manage their discomfort at bedtime, you will be positioning them well for a lifetime of strong mental health and well-being.

Mastery of these parenting and child coping skills will set your child up for greater confidence and competence in independently handling all sorts of difficult situations both day and night. Thus, *Banish Bedtime Battles* addresses child sleep problems within a larger context, one that permits the transference of skills from bedtime to daytime, in support of well-adjusted, competent, and independent children.

We offer a well-researched, time-honored, and effective method for getting children to sleep in their own beds without a battle. Behavioral treatments (i.e., interventions which aim to change child behaviors) are the first-line treatment for sleep problems and are implemented by parents rather than sleep specialists, putting the power in your hands! Bedtime routines, positive reinforcement for behaviors that support sleep, elimination of behaviors that interfere with sleep, parent education, and the development of strong sleep habits are all typical elements of sleep interventions. We will provide information and instruction in each of these domains. Behavioral interventions, such as *Banish Bedtime Battles*, have been found to decrease children's time to fall asleep, reduce the number of nighttime awakenings, improve children's daytime behavior, and give parents a needed break!

We have over thirty years of combined experience working with families and have used this step-by-step formula countless times and with great success. There is one caveat: you must be committed to seeing this through to the end. Otherwise, there will be a low likelihood of success, and even worse, the next attempt to get your child to sleep in their own bed will be all the more difficult. Consider starting the process when your schedule is flexible or has some slack in it. There is no perfect time to start, but we want to reduce the parental strain as much as possible. This may be hard for you too. Making changes to a child's bedtime routine is particularly challenging because it happens at the end of the day when everyone involved is feeling tired and drained. Yet now you can have confidence that it's worth the trouble because you have this book to guide you. The going can be tough, but the destination is ultimately rewarding for you and your child! This six-week plan is composed of parts designed to be completed on a weekly basis. Each part is designed to fit into your busy lifestyle and can be completed in an hour or less.

Supplemental worksheets and resources can be accessed by scanning the QR code below or by going to https://www. highperformance-parenting.com/bbb-appendices.

Everything You Need to Know about Child Sleep

APPROXIMATELY 25–40 PERCENT OF ALL CHILDREN EXPERIENCE sleep problems at some point during childhood.[1] The COVID-19 pandemic led to significant disruptions in child sleep, and the long-term effects of this disruption are yet to be seen. Suffice it to say that you are not alone. Odds are you have at least one child in your household that could benefit from more and better-quality sleep. We'll bet that you could too!

One of the following scenarios may be a good depiction of what happens in your home:

- You lay down with your child in their bed until they (and, quite possibly, you too) have fallen asleep.
- Your child won't sleep unless you're nearby (e.g., working, watching TV, reading) while your child goes to sleep, regardless of whether you want to be there or not.
- Your child falls asleep in your bed (with you in it or nearby).
- Your child falls asleep elsewhere in the home and is carried to bed.

- Preferring to be near to you, especially at night, your child fights tooth and nail to delay going to bed and, once in bed, yells out frequently for you to return. The time from getting into bed to actual sleep sometimes takes hours.

- Your child has difficulty settling down for the evening— just when you've tucked them in, they're out of bed, wandering around.

- You submit to your child's demands to prevent the crying and tantrums that would wake others nearby.

- Your child refuses to get in bed and nightly arguments and unpleasantness ensue.

- Your child willingly goes to sleep in their own bed but wanders into your bedroom at some point during the night. You sometimes don't even wake up when your child climbs into bed with you.

- Your child wakes up at night and calls out repeatedly (or makes a lot of noise!) until you enter your child's room.

- Instead of falling asleep, your child calls out for a drink of water, just one more kiss and hug, to be walked to the bathroom, or just about anything else!

- Your child can fall asleep only if a certain movie, song, or other sounds are present.

- Your child adheres to their bedtime routine so rigidly that if they are even a minute behind schedule, they become emotional.

- Any combination of the above (or similar scenarios) on any given night.

The bedtime battles you've been facing may have been in place since your child was a toddler, or perhaps they began after a stressful life event or illness. It's possible the pattern began because there really is no greater parenting joy than lying down at night, snuggling with your child, chatting, and storytelling. But, as your child has grown older, your expectations for them (and perhaps your own needs) have changed, though your bedtime routine may not have. Whatever the reason for your current battles, you have made the decision to require your child to go to sleep independently.

Notice that most of the listed bedtime scenarios involve you, the parent! It's no wonder that a recent study found that a parent's presence at bedtime is one factor that predicts child sleep problems.[2] The good news about this is that it means you have power to resolve the bedtime battles at hand simply by changing *your* behavior. This book aims to help you determine how to spend the right amount of time with your child at bedtime—enough to support your parent-child connection, but not so much that it will contribute to bedtime problems.

When Ellen's firstborn was only weeks old, her sister-in-law gave her some sage advice: don't do anything one night with your kids that you're not willing to do *every* night. She followed this advice with few deviations, and her sleep (and her children's sleep) enjoyed the benefits of that important parenting tip! Children crave repetition and parental attention. Bedtime routines offer them both, and children will take every second of time and attention they can reasonably eke out of you. These bedtime routines, good or bad, are thus easily established. The good news is, however, that what is learned can also be unlearned. Children are incredibly adaptable and resilient. Once you, as parent, have made your decision clear to your child, and you begin to follow the steps in this book, your child will adapt. They will gain new behaviors, insights, and coping skills, and you will gain some sleep.

Sleep Basics and Foundational Practices

How much do you *really* know about sleep? Understanding a few sleep facts will both demonstrate the importance of sleep and strengthen your commitment to ensuring that you and your child get enough. Sleep problems are at the root of many childhood difficulties because sleep is essential for good physical, cognitive, and social functioning. Once you know how crucial sleep is to healthy functioning, it's much easier to prioritize a good night's sleep.

Sleep is guided by two biological mechanisms that work together to determine when you sleep and when you wake up. One is known as sleep-wake homeostasis (or sleep drive). This is an automatic process that constantly monitors your need for sleep. You are under the influence of this process when you feel an increased need for sleep the longer you are awake. For example, you may feel tired at 11 p.m. but utterly exhausted and unable to keep your eyes open by 2 a.m. The longer you are awake, the stronger your sleep drive (the need and desire for sleep).

The other biological mechanism at work determining when you sleep and when you are awake is known as circadian rhythm. Circadian rhythm is responsible for several bodily functions across a 24-hour cycle. It's what makes you feel alert in the morning and tired at night.

It's very difficult to fight your circadian rhythm. Anyone who's experienced jet lag while traveling can attest to that. When your sleep is in sync with your circadian rhythm, you wake from sleep feeling rested and restored. When your sleep is out of sync, as when you are jet-lagged, your sleep is of lesser quality, even if you get your usual number of hours of sleep. The timing of your sleep is just as important as the number of hours you get. Moreover, sleep that happens in one solid uninterrupted chunk of time is of higher quality than sleep that is made up of smaller periods of sleep, even if the same number of sleep hours are attained in the end. Therefore, we want to prioritize sleep that is in sync with circadian rhythms and gained within one solid chunk of time.[3]

Even though the circadian rhythm operates automatically and out of your awareness, your behavior and environment influence it. Environmental factors such as light and temperature influence the circadian rhythm and can be altered to optimize sleep. We'll discuss how to modify your child's sleeping environment to best support quality sleep in Week 3.

Let's take a closer look at what happens during your child's sleep. Your child cycles through four distinct stages of sleep, plus a stage known as rapid eye movement (REM) sleep. Sleep stages one to four are often referred to as non-REM sleep.

Stages one and two (light sleep): Shortly after your child falls asleep, they drift into a light sleep during which they can easily be awakened. Within five to ten minutes, your child is fully asleep. Your child spends about thirty minutes in these two stages before moving into deep sleep.

Stages three and four (deep sleep): As your child shifts into deep sleep, they become more difficult to be awakened, body movements are minimal, and their muscles are relaxed. These phases of sleep are important for restfulness and their body's restoration. During deep sleep, their body repairs muscles and tissues, stimulates growth, boosts immune function, and builds up energy for the next day.

Rapid eye movement (REM) sleep: Within about ninety minutes of falling asleep, your child enters REM sleep. During this phase, dreaming occurs, your child's eyes dart rapidly back and forth under their closed eyelids (hence the name of the phase) and, although your child's heart rate, breathing, and blood pressure increase, their muscles become paralyzed. This muscle paralysis helps to explain why many children report dreams about being unable to move or escape a situation. It is likely that, though asleep, they have become aware of their inability to move. Each REM period typically lasts from minutes to an hour during which your child's brain processes information from throughout the day, permitting those events to be stored in long-term memory.

Your child moves through the sleep stages in a sequential fashion with more non-REM sleep occurring in the earlier part of the night and more REM sleep in the later part. This explains why your child may wake in the morning in the midst of a dream.

Childhood Sleep Disorders

Children's sleep problems often have multiple causes and can present in a variety of different ways. Many times, these problems are behavioral in nature and can be addressed with the plan as presented in this book (see Behavioral Insomnia below). Other times, a child's sleeping problems may be caused or exacerbated by a physiologically based sleep disorder. Keep in mind, too, that there are a variety of other medical conditions (e.g., asthma, obesity, eczema, acid reflux, anxiety, depression) which can negatively impact sleep.

Approximately 4 percent of children have diagnosable sleep disorders.[4] If you suspect that your child is experiencing a sleep disorder, or if your child's medical condition is negatively impacting their sleep, please consult with your child's doctor. They may refer your child to a sleep medicine specialist who can, if needed, conduct a sleep study, an overnight stay in a sleep laboratory to evaluate your child's sleep in a controlled environment. We'll review some common sleep disorders here.

Behavioral Insomnia

If your child suffers from behavioral insomnia, believe me, you'll know it. Behavioral insomnia involves a child who is very resistant to bedtime, experiences much difficulty falling asleep, or awakens multiple times during the night. The disorder affects approximately 10–30 percent of all children.[5] Behavioral insomnias are often divided into (1) limit-setting insomnia and (2) sleep onset association insomnia.

- *Limit-setting insomnia* involves a child who refuses to go to sleep at their designated bedtime. The child may stall for time, demand to continue with preferred activities, and outright refuse parental requests, pleas, and demands. The refusal may be prolonged enough that the result is sleep loss. The origins of this type of insomnia often involve a lack of limit setting or inconsistent implementation of the bedtime routine by parents.

- *Sleep onset association insomnia* is present when a child is unable to sleep unless certain conditions are present (e.g., parent presence at bedside, TV is turned on for background noise, child's back is rubbed). If the child wakes during the night, the child is unable to fall back to sleep without the presence of the required conditions.

Recommended interventions for behavioral insomnias involve both a behavioral approach and parent education. This six-week plan is specifically designed for children with behavioral insomnia, including limit-setting and sleep onset association insomnias. Our approach is consistent with treatment recommendations which call for behavioral interventions (e.g., bedtime routines, planned ignoring, positive reinforcement) to promote positive child behavior change along with parenting best practices. So if you suspect that your child is suffering from behavioral insomnia, you've got the right book in your hands.

Parasomnias

Parasomnias are sleep disorders that occur when a person is somewhere between asleep and fully awake. The person may appear to be alert and oriented, even walking and talking, but their brain is not entirely awake. They are likely in the midst of a transition from one stage of sleep (stage three or stage four) and wakefulness, suspended somewhere in between, and unlikely to recall the episode once awake.[6] These disorders can occur at any age but are most common in childhood. Ninety-six percent of parasomnias will resolve by early adulthood.[7] They are not thought of as dangerous. Rather, the main concern regards the person's potential to unknowingly harm themselves or someone else during the episode. Parasomnias include, but are not limited to, confusional arousal, sleepwalking, sleep terrors, nightmare disorder, and bedwetting. In the interest of time and readability, we will only review these most common parasomnias here.

- *Confusional arousal.* Children with confusional arousal often show behaviors that are somewhat like sleepwalking or sleep terrors, only milder. The child may sit up in bed with their eyes open, cry out, thrash around, and appear confused. They may be agitated and utter a few words as well. They are often difficult to console, and parent attempts at reassurance may backfire, resulting in increased distress. The episodes typically occur in the first two to three hours of sleep and can last from ten to thirty minutes. In the morning, the child has no recollection of the episode.

- *Sleepwalking.* Almost half of all children aged four to sixteen have experienced sleepwalking.[8] Sleepwalking often starts as confusional arousal but becomes sleepwalking once the child gets out of bed. Children who sleepwalk may quietly walk around the room or the house, appearing to be awake, but "out of it." It's not uncommon to hear a parent report that they were awakened to the sight of their sleepwalking child standing quietly at their bedside. Less frequently, the sleepwalking child may appear agitated or distressed, running through the house. It is important to note that a sleepwalking child can unlock a door and leave the house or perform other potentially dangerous behaviors (e.g., starting the microwave or stove, opening a second-story window) so safety precautions may be warranted. Parents' attempts to talk to the sleepwalker are often met with silence. As with the other parasomnias, sleepwalking typically occurs in the first third of the night and tends to improve as the child gets older.

- *Sleep terrors.* Sleep terrors, also known as night terrors, can be really frightening to a parent. Several hours after the child has fallen asleep, they begin loudly screaming. They may be shaking, trembling, sweating, heart pounding, and appear very scared. They are both inconsolable and nonresponsive to attempts to comfort them. Sleep terrors differ from nightmares in that a child awakens following a nightmare and is often able to recall the details of the bad dream. Frequently following the nightmare, the child becomes reluctant to go to sleep due to fear of recurrent nightmares. The child who experiences a sleep terror is not awake and cannot recall the episode in the morning. Additionally, sleep terrors occur in the first half of the night, and nightmares tend to occur in the second half.

- *Nightmare disorder.* Nightmares are common and rarely cause for concern. They tend to first surface in children between ages three and six and then become less frequent after the age of ten. Girls appear to have nightmares more frequently than boys. If the nightmares are repeated and intense and result in your child's reluctance to go to sleep, sleep disruption, fear or anxiety, or impairments in daytime functioning, your child may be experiencing nightmare disorder. If your child's sleep and daytime functioning are affected by nightmares, it's worth mentioning the problem to your child's doctor.

- *Bedwetting.* Also known as nocturnal enuresis, bedwetting is one of the most frequent sleep problems in childhood, affecting up to 20 percent of school-aged children.[9] The problem typically affects more boys than girls, and a family history of bedwetting is common. The effect on children and families can be quite distressing. Children may experience negative impacts on self-esteem as well as their relationships with parents. Embarrassment about bedwetting may lead children to miss out on sleepovers and other overnight stays. If your child does not have daytime wetting problems, a bedwetting alarm (also referred to as a bell-and-pad alarm) is an effective way to treat the problem.[10] Bedwetting alarms consist of a moisture sensor that is clipped to the child's underwear and an alarm that rings when the sensor detects wetness. With a few weeks of use, the child learns to wake to (rather than sleep through) the sensation of a full bladder, enabling them to use the bathroom. Prescription medications are likely to show more immediate results; yet bedwetting often returns once the medication is stopped. Bedwetting alarms appear to demonstrate more lasting effects[11] and are easily available online.

Sleep-Related Movement Disorders

Sleep-related movement disorders include restless leg syndrome and periodic limb movement disorder. Children with restless leg syndrome may appear fidgety, restless, and complain of sensations such as "tingles" or "spiders" in their legs. Discomfort is experienced by the persistent urge to move one or, more typically, both legs. Symptoms have been found to be associated with low iron, but given the potential for iron toxicity, see your child's doctor before administering iron supplements to your child on your own. Children with restless leg syndrome may also experience periodic limb movement disorder, and both disorders appear to show some association with attention-deficit hyperactivity disorder.[12] Periodic limb movement disorder involves brief jerky movements in the legs or arms during sleep that occur with some regularity (e.g., twenty- to forty-second intervals). Your child might not be aware of the movements, but a parent or sibling might notice it.

Sleep-Related Breathing Disorders

Obstructive sleep apnea occurs in 1–5 percent of children and is caused by obstruction of the upper airway, often caused by large adenoids or tonsils.[13] Treatment often consists of their removal by a procedure known as an adenotonsillectomy. Obstructive sleep apnea is also associated with snoring, bedwetting, unusual sleep positions (e.g., neck bent backward), and morning headaches.

Circadian Rhythm Sleep Disorders

Delayed sleep phase syndrome occurs when a person's start of sleep is delayed by two or more hours. For example, an adolescent might fall asleep at 12:00 or 1:00 a.m. rather than a parent's preferred time of 10:00 p.m. Morning wake times are also delayed by the corresponding number of hours. This syndrome is most characteristic of adolescents, affecting approximately 7–16 percent of teens.[14] This circadian rhythm shift has led researchers to investigate the positive impact of delaying school start times to account for the circadian rhythm shift and allow for more sleep. Research is highly suggestive of many beneficial outcomes (e.g., academic performance, physical and mental health) when the school start time is delayed to 8:30 a.m. or later for middle and high school students, even when that delay nets only a few extra minutes of sleep. Even the addition of a few extra minutes has been demonstrated to translate into improved functioning. Research consistently demonstrates improvements in sleep durations, school attendance rates, grade point averages, achievement scores, attention levels, and physical and mental health when school start times are delayed.[15] See the American Academy of Sleep Medicine position statement at https://aasm.org/advocacy/position-statements/delaying-school-start-times-student-health/ for more information on school start times.

HOW MUCH SLEEP SHOULD MY CHILD GET?

To answer this question, let's turn to the sleep experts. Table 1.1 presents the recommended hours of sleep for children as suggested by the National Sleep Foundation.[16]

These numbers are intended to serve as guidelines. The number of hours of sleep that your child needs depends upon factors

Table 1.1. National Sleep Foundation's Recommended Hours of Sleep by Child Age

	Age Range	Recommended Hours of Sleep
Newborn	0–3 months	14–17 hours
Infant	4–11 months	12–15 hours
Toddler	1–2 years	11–14 hours
Preschool	3–5 years	10–13 hours
School-age	6–13 years	9–11 hours
Teen	14–17 years	8–10 hours
Young Adult	18–25 years	7–9 hours
Adult	26–64 years	7–9 hours
Older Adult	65 or more years	7–8 hours

that are unique to your child, such as activity level and health status. In short, the right amount of sleep is what makes your child feel good and function well.

Not getting enough sleep is quite common among middle and high school–aged children and adolescents. Typical school start times (e.g., 7:15 a.m.) are inconsistent with the biological needs of this age group. As children enter puberty, their circadian rhythms naturally shift toward getting sleepy later at night and, thus, needing to wake up later in the mornings. The American Academy of Pediatrics recently recommended that middle and high school start times are set no earlier than 8:30 a.m. to provide students the opportunity to get the sleep they need.

Not only is the amount of sleep important, but sleep quality matters too. There are many factors (e.g., light exposure, temperature, stress, food) that can influence the quality of your child's sleep. We recommend using this knowledge to your advantage by decreasing or eliminating those factors known to disrupt sleep and increasing those factors that promote sleep. We'll return to this topic in Week 3 when you'll begin to prepare your child's sleep environment.

Consistent Bedtime Routine

Healthy bedtime routines are the bedrock of good sleep. Without them, a child is at high risk for sleep problems. Bedtime routines are those behaviors or practices a child engages in during the time leading up to sleep. These routines may include nutrition (e.g., drink of water, healthy snack), hygiene behaviors (e.g., bathing, washing face, brushing teeth), communication (e.g., book reading, prayer, singing, storytelling), physical contact (e.g., snuggling with your child), and any other family cultural practices.

Daily routines are not just important for sleep but have implications for child development and well-being more generally. Benefits of everyday routines are positive impacts on (1) good self-care and health, (2) literacy and language development, (3) parent and family functioning, (4) emotional and behavioral regulation, *and* (5) sleep.[17] Healthy bedtime routines also pave the way for the development of long-term healthy habits. In short, you can get a lot of bang for no bucks just by having your child follow a bedtime routine. Even better news is that some studies have found intimate partner relationship satisfaction to improve when a consistent bedtime routine is established for the child.[18]

Aim to foster a slow and calming bedtime routine. Nighttime races to put on pajamas, exuberant singing, and energizing videos are stimulating and, therefore, not conducive to easing your child into a restful slumber. Take every opportunity to promote the nighttime conditions that facilitate sleep. One way to do this is to have your child bathe or shower in warm water just before bed, as the body's natural cooling process promotes the onset of sleep.[19] Additionally, gentle massage has also been found to decrease stress hormones (e.g., cortisol) and increase feel-good chemicals in the brain (e.g., serotonin, dopamine), thus helping to reduce the stress and worry that can sometimes prevent one from drifting off.[20] Keep the bedtime routine to thirty minutes or less. If the routine is substantially longer, the result is often a delay in the timing of falling asleep, which translates to less time asleep.

Be sure your child's routine is consistent. Children thrive in environments that are predictable. Knowing the time to start getting ready for bed, the sequence of events in the routine, as well as the time for lights out, helps to avoid those bedtime battles. This organized sequence of events is associated with an earlier bedtime, decreased time to fall asleep, decreased nighttime awakenings, increased time asleep, and, best of all, increased parent sleep quality. Everyone wins! While every family will have to adjust the bedtime routine now and again due to a variety of life circumstances, the key is to be *as consistent as possible* and to avoid needing to change things when first establishing the routine. Consistency *now* allows for a bit of flexibility *later*. A lack of consistency when establishing the routine, however, may send the whole project down the drain (and make it even harder to reestablish the routine later).

SLEEP ENVIRONMENT

Create a sleep environment that is conducive to sleep. Factors that interfere with falling and staying asleep include technology use, light, and noise. When it comes to technology, banish it from the bedroom and bedtime routine whenever possible. A recent study found that children who read a book rather than used an electronic device in the hour before going to sleep had better sleep duration, sleep quality, sleep efficiency, and weight status than those who used an electronic device.[21] Reduce distractions and ensure a quiet and restful sleeping environment.

If your child is afraid of the dark, a single dim night-light is fine; however, avoid an overreliance on the light. Take care not to overly accommodate a child's fear of the dark (Week 2 will present greater detail on accommodation). Dim night-lights can be used initially and phased out once a strong routine and high-quality sleep have been established. Whenever possible, keep the temperature cool (below 72 degrees Fahrenheit) and ensure that your child has blankets for warmth and comfort.

As discussed in the Childhood Sleep Disorders section, children often develop strong sleep associations. This means they may associate falling asleep with the presence of a stuffed animal, a favorite blanket, a pet, or even the presence of a parent or sibling. These associations are sometimes referred to as sleep "crutches" or "props," highlighting the fact that they are generally regarded to be unhelpful, even counterproductive, when used in the long-term. If you've read any other books about helping your child resolve sleep problems, chances are the author endorsed use of a sleep crutch such as a stuffed animal or a night-light. You won't find that suggestion here because we strongly believe that providing a sleep crutch sends the wrong message to the child—one that suggests that you don't think they can sleep on their own and we know they can learn to sleep without it! If a child develops a sleep association that interferes with their ability to sleep on a regular basis, they may meet criteria for sleep onset association insomnia.

To avoid sleep onset association insomnia, be sure that the presence of objects at the onset of sleep are those that (1) promote sleep, (2) can be available each and every night, and (3) don't serve as a "sleep crutch." Recall, too, that independent sleep requires the sleeper to drift off on their own, without the presence or intervention of another person, so be sure that your child is not reliant on the sight, touch (e.g., back rub), or sound (e.g., reading, soft singing) of a person when they fall to sleep.

Additionally, when a child's bedroom (and bed, especially) is used for purposes other than sleeping, that use can interfere with the association between bed and sleep. For example, if your child commonly does homework in bed, they may crawl in at night only to find their mind racing with academic thoughts! Alternatively, if they frequently snack in bed, they might feel hungry just as they curl up under the covers. So limit the use of your child's bed to relaxing and sleeping only.

Using Biology to Your Advantage

Earlier you learned that the circadian rhythm is responsible for several bodily functions including wakefulness across the day and night. That rhythm can be facilitated by doing things that are consistent with the body's natural operations. Take, for example, the influence of light on the human body. Often, we feel tired as soon as daylight dims and darkness takes over. If we were to remain inside in a bright environment with no visual cues of the late hour, we would be likely to feel more alert and awake. Light matters!

Exposure to artificial light at the wrong times can disrupt the body's natural sleep-wake cycle. Many electronic devices (e.g., smart phones, tablets, computer screens, televisions) emit what is known as blue light. Contrary to popular belief, blue light isn't actually bad; what matters is *when* someone is exposed to it. Sunlight, for example, is the main source of blue light and exposure during the morning and daytime helps to promote sleep at night. Blue light boosts mood, attention, energy, and activity levels. Blue light exposure at night, however, interferes with the body's circadian rhythm, tricking it into believing that there is still daylight and making sleep harder to come by, shifting the circadian rhythm by as much as three hours![22] Use of blue light–filtering eyewear, setting blue light–emitting devices to "night mode," and blue light–filtering software may reduce interference with the circadian rhythm, although to date, research is limited. Therefore, it is important to refrain from exposure to blue light in the two to three hours leading up to bedtime.

Sleep Aids

There are many products touted to help one gain a better night's sleep; yet sleep aids are the antithesis of independent sleep. As such, we discourage their use in favor of behavioral strategies which are safe, effective, and well researched.

Over-the-counter sleep aids such as melatonin supplements and sedating antihistamines are commonly taken in pill form with the intent of producing better and longer sleep. Melatonin is a hormone that is produced in the brain and is largely responsible for regulation of the sleep-wake cycle. It is more effective at helping one to fall asleep, rather than stay asleep.

Use of melatonin supplements for children's sleep has increased since the onset of the COVID-19 pandemic despite a lack of high-quality evidence demonstrating its safety. The U.S. Food and Drug Administration does not regulate or approve the use of melatonin supplements. A 2023 *Journal of the American Medical Association* study investigating the quantity of melatonin in pediatric gummies sold in the United States reveals that the actual quantity of melatonin in the products ranged from 74 percent to 347 percent of the labeled quantity! Eighty-eight percent of the products were inaccurately labeled, and one did not contain any melatonin at all.[23] Thus, it is crucial that parents are aware that use of melatonin gummies may result in the ingestion of melatonin vastly different than the labeled quantities. Provided this, it may come as no surprise that phone calls regarding melatonin ingestion made to the U.S. Poison Control Centers increased 530 percent from 2012 to 2021.[24] Use of melatonin supplements, when deemed necessary, should be done in close consultation with your child's doctor.

In recent decades, many parents have resorted to using antihistamines (e.g., Benadryl) to help their children sleep due to their sedating effects. There are some significant downsides to their use, however, such as side effects including headaches and the development of tolerance to the drug so that a child needs more and more of the substance over time to make them sleepy. Additionally, antihistamines tend to leave one feeling groggy the following day (the so-called hangover effect).

Note that there are no prescription medications approved to help children sleep. Sleeping pills come with side effects, haven't been fully tested with children, and have unknown long-term effects. As with any medication, vitamin, or supplement you intend to give to your child, check in with their doctor first. Ask about the drug's benefits, side effects and risks, whether it will really help your child's sleep problem, especially in the long-term, and whether there are other nondrug solutions that may help.

Nondrug options include essential oil aromatherapy (e.g., lavender), weighted blankets, sleep stories (audio stories designed to help the child drift off), and other products. These products have been marketed to promote sleep, and they *can* help achieve more sleep, especially if your child develops an association between the product and the act of falling asleep. Before using such products as sleep aids, however, be aware that if your child develops a reliance on a particular product, it can significantly interfere with their sleep on occasions when they are required to sleep without it (think of sleepovers or other nights spent away from home when the product is unavailable to the child at bedtime). Many children are dependent on a sleep aid (e.g., fan) and this interferes with the child's ability to sleep away from home (or during power outages!). It is best to ensure that your child can sleep both with and without these aids to avoid future problems. With these precautions in mind, these aids can be helpful in the *transition* to independent sleep because they can help your child to be more comfortable and confident as they make important changes to their sleep routines.

In general, these sleep aids should be used on a short-term basis, if at all. Sleep aids cannot overcome bad sleep habits! Lifestyle changes that promote sleep, along with coping skills (presented in Week 3), are the most effective options to sustain good sleeping habits.

Nutrition

There's no doubt about it—nutrition affects sleep. There are foods known to promote sleep and foods known to interfere with it. Sleep-enhancing foods include nuts such as almonds, walnuts, peanuts, and cashews. These nuts contain melatonin and are a significant source of the mineral magnesium. Magnesium appears to assist sleep by reducing inflammation and possibly reducing cortisol, a hormone associated with stress and anxiety. Other foods containing melatonin are milk, rice and other grains (barley, rolled oats), as well as many fruits and vegetables (tart cherries, corn, tomatoes, olives, asparagus, pomegranate, cucumber, broccoli). Try adding some of these to your next grocery list!

Your child should avoid caffeine in the hours leading up to bedtime. Most of us are aware of the presence of caffeine in coffee and soda, but you might be surprised by some of the other foods serving up a good jolt of caffeine—hot cocoa, puddings, cookies, and ice cream are often caffeinated due to having chocolate as an ingredient. Commonly used medications can be surprising sources of caffeine. Check the labels on pain relievers, cold medicines, and even some herbal remedies to determine whether they contain caffeine. Since the effects of caffeine last a while, limit caffeine consumption to morning through late afternoon.

Additionally, high-fat diets have been linked to poor sleep (increased nighttime awakenings, less deep sleep), as well as eating high protein or large meals just before bed. Bodily resources and energy spent on digestion can interfere with your child's ability to sleep. High-sugar foods and refined starches (e.g., white bread, pasta, white rice, pastries) can cause cortisol levels to rise, making sleep harder to achieve; therefore, foods that have a lower impact on blood sugar (e.g., nuts, hard-boiled egg, cheese, fruits, carrots with hummus) are best for bedtime snacking. Missing meals also raises cortisol levels and makes it more difficult to get a restful night's sleep.[25] We've organized the dos and don'ts of evening snacking in table 1.2, which presents foods that either promote or interfere with sleep. Keep in mind that while these nutrition recommendations are presented for children, they will be of benefit to parents as well! Before making significant dietary changes, however, it's best to consult with your child's doctor.

Table 1.2. Foods That Promote Sleep or Interfere with Sleep

Foods That Promote Sleep	Foods That Interfere with Sleep
Nuts (almonds, walnuts, pistachios)	Sugary beverages (sodas)
Lean proteins (turkey, fish)	Sugary treats (soda, candy, high-sugar cereals, doughnuts)
Dairy products (milk, yogurt, cottage cheese)	Caffeinated foods (chocolate)
Hummus	Caffeinated beverages (coffee, tea)
Tart cherry juice	High-fat foods (pizza, fries, ice cream)
Fruits (kiwi, figs, prunes, bananas)	Spicy foods (hot sauce, curries)
Vegetables (corn, olives, cucumber)	Highly acidic foods (oranges, grapefruits, tomatoes)
Rice and grains (barley, rolled oats)	
Herbal teas (chamomile, passionflower, lemon balm)	

In short, a healthy diet is best for achieving a good night's sleep. Sleep can be affected by missing necessary nutrients and, therefore, improved by a healthy diet and the use of dietary supplements, such as vitamins, minerals, and micronutrients.

A final note about those middle-of-the-night "I'm hungry" declarations some of you might hear from your child. A child six years of age or older who routinely eats a healthy diet is unlikely to experience true hunger-related, middle-of-the-night waking. So you can be assured, it's okay to send them back to bed without the snack.

EXERCISE

Regular physical activity improves sleep. U.S. Department of Health and Human Services exercise guidelines recommend that children have at least sixty minutes of moderate to vigorous physical activity (e.g., brisk walking, running) daily, but *even as little as ten minutes of daily aerobic activity can yield great sleep-promoting benefits.*[26] In a European study on childhood sleep patterns, researchers found that, in a sample of 591 seven-year-old children, the average time to fall asleep was twenty-six minutes. Approximately one out of ten children had difficulty falling asleep and took about fifteen minutes longer than the other children. The researchers also noticed that children who were more physically active during the day took less time to fall asleep at night. They discovered that every hour of sedentary activity during the day was associated with an additional three minutes to fall asleep.[27]

Because exercising produces endorphins (euphoria-inducing chemicals) and raises body temperature, both of which make it harder to fall asleep, it's best to avoid exercise four to five hours before bedtime.

CHILD DEVELOPMENT

Children's sleep requirements change over time as they grow and develop. This means that their bedtime routines need to change as well. One of the tricky parts of being a parent is knowing when it's time to level-up your parenting. We've worked with plenty of parents of school-aged children whose bedtime routines haven't changed since their children were toddlers! We know it's not always clear when it's time to upgrade the routine, but we'd like to make one thing clear: school-aged children can be terrific at going to sleep on their own! They *do not* need their parents to lie with them at bedtime until they drift off to sleep. Any initial upset at a new bedtime routine that is less dependent on parents and more reliant on their own independence will be short-lived. Kids thrive on doing things on their own. The sense of accomplishment is tremendously rewarding.

Sometimes we get questions from parents who are concerned about the emotional toll that crying and distress at bedtime may have on their child. The research is quite clear on this. Behavioral sleep techniques such as those described in this book do not have harmful impacts on children's emotions, behaviors, parent-child relationships, or psychosocial functioning.[28] Any periods of crying or distress will not be harmful to your child. Distressing in the moment? Yes, but not harmful. In fact, failing to support and encourage your child's independence can have significant negative effects on their emotional and behavioral functioning. Children who don't believe in themselves are children who often fail to set appropriate goals for themselves, unsure of whether they can achieve them on their own. Children who learn that they can do things autonomously are those that thrive.

Choosing the Bedtime Routine

The bedtime routine that you and your child develop will be unique but should contain the following elements: nutrition, hygiene behaviors, communication, and physical contact. This week, you'll decide on the specific set of activities that your child will engage in each night leading up to bedtime using the Ideal Bedtime Routine worksheet. See one example of a child's ideal bedtime routine in figure 1.1. Seek the input of your child as you set the bedtime routine because doing so will cement their commitment and make those bedtime battles less likely to occur. As you consult with your child, make sure not to agree to anything that cannot be implemented consistently. You, as your child's parent, know what is in their best interest! Avoid the temptation to give in to your child's requests for bedtime routines that are not conducive to sleep, require too much of your effort to implement, or are overly indulgent.

The routines that are the smoothest and most successful are those that can be carried out each night without much deviation. That means that your routine shouldn't be too long. If it is, there are too many opportunities for the routine to get off track. On the other hand, the routine should be long enough to allow your child's body and mind to wind down and prepare for sleep to come. Aim for a routine that's approximately thirty minutes.

As you make decisions about your child's bedtime routine, keep in mind that it's essential that you stick with these decisions, so choose them with an eye toward what you think you'll be able to do consistently. Remember, we are not asking you to implement this plan just yet! We just want you to begin to draft the plan. The kick-off of the plan will come later in Week 5.

You already have these bedtime routine elements in place, you say? Excellent, but it's a great idea to revisit the routine to ensure that it's the best that it can be. Does it need updating as your child has grown older? Are there parts of the routine that might be tweaked to enhance your child's compliance? Does the routine contain all of the elements of an ideal routine? Use the Current Bedtime Routine and Ideal Bedtime Routine worksheets referenced below to set you and your child up for success. Weeks 2–6 will present guidance on how to make the routine *effective* for your child and your family!

Ideal Bedtime Routine

Date:
7/28/24

Design your child's ideal bedtime routine. For each evening hour, list your child's ideal bedtime activities in the chart below. Be sure to design a plan that you can apply consistently.

Time	Ideal Bedtime Activity:	Remember to Include :
7:45 pm	Isabella eats a healthy snack in the kitchen.	✓ Nutrition (healthy bedtime snack, drink)
8:00 pm	Isabella puts on pajamas in bedroom. Washes face and brushes teeth in bathroom. Uses toilet.	✓ Hygiene behaviors (tooth brushing, washing) ✓ Communication (singing, reading, storytelling)
8:10 pm	We read two books (Isabella chooses one. I choose one) on the couch in the living room. TV is off.	✓ Physical contact (snuggling, massaging) ☐ Other:
8:20 pm	I give Isabella a quick back rub while we talk on the couch. All electronic devices are off.	**Remember to Remove/Reduce:** ✓ Technology ✓ Light
8:30 pm	I give one kiss and hug goodnight and then Isabella goes to bedroom and gets in bed on her own.	✓ Noise ✓ Room Temperature
8:35 pm	Isabella stays in her bed until morning.	**Recommended Hours of Sleep** 0-3 mos. ⟶ 14-17 hrs.
: pm		4-11 mos. ⟶ 12-15 hrs. 1-2 yrs. ⟶ 11-14 hrs.
: pm		3-5 yrs. ⟶ 10-13 hrs. 6-13 yrs. ⟶ 9-11 hrs.
: pm		14-17 yrs. ⟶ 8-10 hrs.

NOTES:

Snack ideas: nuts, hard boiled egg, cheese, fruit, carrots with hummus.

Be consistent each night! Keep the routine short and sweet, and praise the behaviors that I want to see.

Figure 1.1. Sample Ideal Bedtime Routine. *Source:* High Performance Parenting (www.highperformance-parenting.com)

Now Apply It!

1. Document your child's current bedtime routine using the Current Bedtime Routine worksheet.*

2. In consultation with your child, design your child's ideal bedtime routine using the Ideal Bedtime Routine worksheet.* Remember: don't agree to anything that cannot be implemented consistently. Avoid the temptation to give in to your child's requests for bedtime routines that are not conducive to sleep, require too much of your effort to implement, or are overly indulgent. It's not time to implement this plan just yet! You are only in the drafting stage. The plan's kick-off will come later in Week 5.

*Access the worksheets by scanning the QR code below or by going to www.highperformance-parenting .com/bbb-appendices.

WEEK 1 SUMMARY

- Many children struggle to fall and stay asleep. You are not alone!

- Sleep is guided by the circadian rhythm, which operates automatically, but can be influenced by environmental factors (e.g., light and temperature).

- There are four stages of sleep that last about ninety minutes before entering REM sleep.

- There are numerous sleep disorders that can occur in childhood. If you suspect your child has a sleep disorder other than behavioral insomnia, talk to your child's doctor. If you believe that your child has behavioral insomnia, you've got the right book! Our approach follows the recommended strategy for treating this disorder.

- Key elements of sleep interventions for children include bedtime routines, positive reinforcement for behaviors that support sleep, elimination of behaviors that interfere with sleep, parent education, and development of strong sleep habits.

- Bedtime routines need to be calm and consistent. A strong bedtime routine typically includes nutrition, hygiene behaviors, communication, and physical contact. These elements will be specific to your own family.

- Technology use, light, and noise interfere with the sleeping environment and make it harder to fall and stay asleep.

- Beware of the potential for your child to develop strong sleep associations, requiring the presence of a certain stuffed animal, sibling, parent, or pet to fall asleep. In order to establish independent sleep, the child must be able to sleep without another person (e.g., parent, sibling), object (e.g., stuffed animal, night-light), or action (e.g., back rubs, reading).

- Over-the-counter sleep aids (e.g., melatonin supplements, antihistamines) are discouraged and should be used only in consultation with your child's doctor. Research has shown that these sleep aids have limited effectiveness. Furthermore, the quantity of melatonin in melatonin gummies may be vastly different that the labeled amounts, leading to unpredictable amounts ingested by a child.

- Nondrug sleep aids (e.g., lavender oil, a weighted blanket) may be helpful in the short-term. However, when used long-term, your child can develop a counterproductive reliance on the products.

- Caffeine can be sneaky. This substance can be found in sweets containing chocolate, as well as some pain relievers, cold medicines, and herbal remedies. Carefully check for caffeine in the foods your child is eating close to bedtime.

- Exercise during the day is important for health and promotes restful sleep.

Parenting

What's Your Style?

AS PARENTS, YOU HAVE A LOT ON YOUR PLATE. YOU ARE EXPECTED to be familiar with child development, both physical and emotional, and be skilled in parenting. Add in the minutia of other parenting responsibilities (from packing school lunches to helping with math homework), and you've got a lot to manage! We are here to help. This week, we are going to cover some basics about children's emotional functioning and offer some support in finding the style of parenting that gets the results you want.

MAKE WAY FOR EMOTIONS

First-time expectant parents often have a good sense of how their infant will behave. There's cuddling, cooing, feeding, sleeping, a lot of crying, and diapering needs. This is not to say that new parents have it easy. They don't! But in general, they know what to expect and an infant's behavioral repertoire is pretty limited. Then those infants grow into toddlers and their behaviors change drastically. They suddenly become mobile, have preferences, and start to express those preferences, usually in the form of "No!" Parents wade further into uncharted territory here and hope that toddlerhood will give way to more reason, agreeableness, and independence.

If you're reading this, you likely have a school-aged child. Are they more reasonable, agreeable, and independent than they were as toddlers? Objectively, yes. But there's probably a long way to go. "School age" refers to a wide range of ages (five to thirteen), but, in general, your child is at a stage of development in which life is becoming more complex. Their activities are no longer limited to playdates and naps, feeding and potty training. They are learning through play and work, honing their language skills, exploring their identity and sense of autonomy, as well as learning how the world works. Now add in social complexities that school brings ("Asha called me a name today," "Other kids got the answer right, and I got it wrong"), homework, and responsibilities or chores at home.

In thinking about all these new experiences, interests, and concerns, your child experiences strong emotions, which motivate them to seek feel-good experiences and avoid unpleasant experiences. This is in their hardwiring, and it's something we adults do too. We enjoy the taste of a new food and immediately we're motivated to eat more of it. We feel frustrated while waiting in a long line at the grocery store, and we're motivated to return at a different time of day on future trips (or avoid the store altogether).

The difference between children expressing their emotions and adults expressing their emotions is that adults have, for the most part, developed emotion regulation strategies, or coping skills, that help them control the intensity of their emotions and express them in relatively productive and socially acceptable ways. Take the grocery store example. Most adults who feel frustrated waiting in a long line are not going to start crying and stomping their feet. They use emotion regulation skills to cope with that frustration such as considering the relative size of the problem (small), taking deep breaths, and problem-solving. However, children aren't born with these skills. They learn them over the course of years (even decades), so during the school-age years, you should expect a great deal of emotional dysregulation as they learn how to self-regulate.

Let's examine what happens when a child has an experience and lacks emotional coping skills to effectively navigate it. Children experience an event, that experience is filtered through their individual understanding of it, and an emotion is generated to help them either move in the direction of the feel-good experience or away from an unpleasant one. This system, designed to promote survival and well-being, seems reasonable, right? Well, this system hits a snag when circumstances don't allow the child to move in the instinctive and desired direction.

Here's an example. If a child is watching their favorite TV show, they feel happy and this happiness motivates them to keep watching in order to maintain that feel-good experience. Then the parent comes along and says that it's time for bed and they must turn off the TV (system snag) and the child feels frustrated. The child *without* coping skills is likely to express that emotion by way of a tantrum in an effort to keep that feel-good experience going. The child *with* coping skills quickly takes an alternate perspective ("I'll watch again tomorrow," "I'm tired anyway") or even problem-solves by asking the parent for permission to finish watching the last five minutes of the TV show. You might be wondering how to help your child develop such coping skills. The good news is that you're part of the way there already!

Humans experience emotions to drive them to engage in adaptive behaviors. Let's say one feels happy. The feeling of happiness increases the odds one will repeat whatever action or inaction brought about that happiness, thus resulting in more happiness. Feeling sad often promotes human connection needed to get through challenges; feeling scared leads to heightened awareness and caution, even escape from danger. Emotions are not just common human experiences, they're key to survival. If humans never experienced emotions, it's likely that we would have gone extinct long ago.

Now that you're armed with the knowledge about the function of your child's emotions, you're in a better position to help your child. Parents don't always see a child's expression of emotion for what it is—a healthy and natural child behavior. Parents often interpret it through their own biased lenses, which can include beliefs such as "My child shouldn't get upset," "If my child is upset, it means I'm a bad parent," "My child's emotions are too overwhelming for them," or "I'm okay only if my child feels okay." These types of beliefs may have roots way back in a parent's childhood because of *their* parents' modeling or society's messaging about how children *should* behave. Whatever the origins of the beliefs, it's important to understand that children have emotions and need to be able to express them in order to develop healthy lifelong coping skills. Next, we'll look at how parents tend to respond to their child's emotions and behaviors, also known as parenting style.

You've Got Style

A parenting style is the way that a parent relates to their child and responds to their child's behavior. This book assumes that you generally parent your child with love, care, and heart-felt good intentions. The way that parents *show* their love, care, and heart-felt good intentions differs, of course.

Parenting practices and values differ across cultures. Optimal parenting styles, as well as optimal child sleep patterns, should take cultural and community values into consideration. Some families may prioritize time with family, leading to longer or later dinners and possibly later bedtimes. Other cultures may place more emphasis on academic success and, thus, are more permissive of studying during the evening hours. We encourage you to consider that healthy sleep recommendations may not generalize to all cultural groups nor to all individuals within such groups. With that said, we want to be very clear that sufficient sleep is a human need, regardless of one's cultural background. So as you consider your family's needs, parenting style, and cultural practices and beliefs, please regard your child's sleep as something of great importance to your child's well-being, mental health, and optimal functioning. There is no child, regardless of culture, who is at their best without plenty of sleep.

Your parenting style directly affects your child's development, including their bedtime and sleep habits. Parenting styles typically fall into one of four main types, though parents may occasionally switch from one style to another when the situation calls for it. In U.S. culture, there is one type of parenting style that is best for supporting healthy child development and family functioning, which we will guide you toward. As you read through the four styles of parenting, see if you can guess which one it is.

No Nonsense Parenting

First up is No Nonsense parenting, a style characterized by sternness. This style of parenting is low in warmth (sensitivity to and acknowledgment of the child's emotional experience) and high in firmness (follow-through with expectations for child behavior). A No Nonsense parent is demanding and "rules with an iron fist," dominating the child without much regard for the child's feelings, preferences, or experiences. "My way or the highway" comes to mind. How it plays out: if a child expresses a desire for the parent to read just one more book at bedtime, the No Nonsense parent says, "I don't care what you want. Just go to sleep." As a result, the child will likely be obedient but may also develop issues with self-esteem, have hostility toward the parent, and may go on to engage in rebellious behavior.

This style of parenting is often a natural reaction to the confusing, frustrating, and downright annoying behaviors that children can sometimes show, especially at bedtime when everyone is feeling tired. When children repeatedly misbehave, No Nonsense parents often accelerate their efforts to gain control (e.g., yelling). In extreme cases, the No Nonsense parenting behaviors can become abusive.

Once the No Nonsense parent ratchets up a demanding attitude to an intolerable degree, the child submits to the parent's demands. Unfortunately, a vicious cycle can result in which (1) the child is compliant only when the parent becomes angry and (2) the parent escalates their demands for compliance because it resulted in child compliance in the past. Thus, both parent and child behaviors are reinforced, and the pattern continues. If this sounds like you, have no fear. When one party (parent or child) breaks the cycle (for example, a parent makes a clear and direct request of the child while remaining calm), the child is more likely to respond positively to the parent's request. Child compliance may not be immediate once the old pattern is broken, but with patience and consistency, a new and healthier pattern can be developed.

You're On Your Own Parenting

You're On Your Own parenting, a style of parenting low in both warmth and firmness, is best characterized by an absent or unresponsive parent who relies on the child to more or less raise themselves. This parent has a laissez-faire approach in which few limits are set for the child and communication between parent and child is limited. Children of You're On Your Own parents may learn to be resilient and self-sufficient given their need to take care of themselves. Yet this type of parenting has been demonstrated to lead to children who have a hard time controlling their emotions, struggle in academic and social settings, and develop fewer coping skills.[1] How it plays out: the child doesn't ask for an extra book at bedtime because the You're On Your Own parent doesn't do any tuck-ins or bedtime reading in the first place. Certainly, no one sets out to be a You're On Your Own parent—this style of parenting may arise as a result of extreme parental stress or distress, or giving less priority to parenting, sometimes by sheer necessity. By the way, a parent who takes the time to read a parenting book to improve their child and family's functioning is demonstrating highly *involved* parenting!

Anything Goes Parenting

Next up is Anything Goes parenting, a style high in warmth but low in firmness. An Anything Goes parent is lenient with the child and rarely follows through on consequences, which can lead to behavioral and emotional problems for the child. How it plays out: the child expresses a desire for the parent to read just one more book at bedtime, the Anything Goes parent says, "Okay, you've got it!" Generally speaking, this is the parenting style that has led to the situation you may be finding yourself in now, in which the child is running the show at bedtime.

When a child expresses that they want to co-sleep with the parent due to a fear of the dark, for example, the Anything Goes parent accommodates this fear and permits co-sleeping even though it's inconvenient, uncomfortable, or against the parent's better judgment. It's what the child wants, after all! Other well-meaning parents might not give in merely to indulge the child but rather out of a desire to reduce their child's distress. The problem with this permissive approach is twofold: (1) the child learns that their fear of the dark is warranted, and they do, in fact, need their parent present to be and feel safe (which often negatively impacts daily functioning outside of bedtime) *and* (2) it makes it very difficult to change your approach when you eventually want to get the child back into their own bed. Furthermore, it may not surprise you to learn that children of Anything Goes parents often tend toward being aggressive, less self-reliant, less able to maintain self-control, and more unhappy.

Anything Goes parents tend to yield to their children's wants, preferences, requests, and demands. Note that accommodating a child's preferences is not inherently bad. *Too much* accommodation, however, leads to problems. Like anything in life, balance is key. If a child prefers vanilla over chocolate, sure, accommodate their preference, because doing so does not lead to future problems (none that we can think of, anyway). Accommodating a school-aged child's preference to sleep with a parent every night, however, does lead to future problems. Other examples include routinely ordering food on behalf of a child who is too timid to voice their own order or limiting the family's restaurant options because they are a finicky eater. Here's a good rule for determining whether your accommodation is problematic or innocuous: if it hinders your child's ability to function *independently* now or in the future (considering their developmental stage), then it's the kind you want to avoid. If the accommodation has the effect of promoting your child's confidence or willingness and ability to face challenges or, at the very least, has a neutral effect on your child's self-reliance, then it's probably okay.

We are specialists in the treatment of anxiety and *accommodation* is a key term in our work. Generally, we see families who have inadvertently been accommodating a child's worry or anxiety, reaching a point where the anxiety has begun interfering with daily functioning and requires intervention. Day in and day out, we recommend to these parents that they deliberately avoid accommodating their child's worries and anxieties, as doing so keeps the anxiety going and, often, makes it worse. For example, if a child has a fear of the dark and wants to use multiple night-lights, does accommodating their fear serve them or hurt them? Well, using the night-lights increases the child's comfort in the short-term but also suggests that the dark is indeed something to be feared. Additionally, the parent inadvertently sends the message that the child can't cope in the dark, undermining the child's self-confidence. Considering that darkness is a natural part of life, children need to believe in their ability to handle the dark and other challenging situations that life throws their way.

Learning and applying this model (e.g., "face your fears to overcome your fears") will enhance your child's self-confidence and lay the foundation for mastering future difficult or scary situations. Helping your child avoid challenging situations (i.e., accommodation) deprives them of critical coping skill practice.

As you can see, Anything Goes parenting does not do children any favors. This type of parenting often brings harmony in the short-term but causes major problems in the long-term and, therefore, is generally not recommended.

Some parents may recognize the term *accommodation* from experience with school-based supports for students with disabilities. Children with medical conditions may require certain accommodations to access a domain such as education. When we write of accommodation here, we are referring to something a bit different. Accommodation here refers to changing what is required of your child in order to remove or prevent mild to moderate anxiety, discomfort, or distress. By not swooping in to "save" your child, it requires them to learn to be independent, ultimately increasing their self-confidence, self-competence, and coping skills, while also reducing anxiety and distress in the long-term.

Balanced (Warm and Firm) Parenting

This leads us to the optimal parenting style—the Balanced parenting style. This style involves both warm and firm parenting, in which the child's feelings are acknowledged and validated *and* parents maintain expectations and deliver consistent consequences. How it plays out: if the child expresses a desire for the parent to read just one more book at bedtime, the Balanced parent says, "You really love story time. Me too (*warm*). But you know the rules, only one story at bedtime (*firm*). Which story do you want to read tomorrow night?" Warm and firm. You are upholding the expectation in a supportive and kind manner and offering encouragement and belief in your child's ability to cope. Another example: a Balanced parent of a child begging to sleep in their parent's bed says, "I know you want to sleep in my bed, but your bed is for you and my bed is for me . . . so you'll be sleeping in your bed. I know you can do it!"

If the child has a history of being permitted to sleep in the parent's bed, however, this is probably not enough to get the child back into their own bed. After all, if it were this easy to undo, this book might end here! The remainder of this book is designed to help you use Balanced parenting skills to get your child sleeping independently.

The Balanced style of parenting promotes positive outcomes for children. Added benefits of this parenting style include improved parent-child relationships, a more peaceful home environment, a more confident child, and a happier parent who is better equipped to handle future parenting challenges.

Balanced parenting features the use of *positive reinforcement* to modify child behaviors. Reward your child (be it with meaningful praise, high fives, tangible rewards, fun activities, etc.) for engaging in the behaviors that you want to see more of (e.g., following directions, facing a fear), in order to increase the likelihood that the behavior will continue in the future.

Meaningful praise and acknowledgment sounds like this:

- You stopped what you were doing right when I asked you to—I noticed!

- You've been brushing your teeth without a reminder—that shows maturity and it's nice to know that I can count on you to be doing your part!

- *(In a whisper)* I saw you sharing that toy with your sister . . . I know she appreciates you.

Notice the specificity in the recognition. Avoid empty praise such as "Good job" and "That's cool" as this is less likely to reinforce the desired behavior.

Positive reinforcement strategies increase desired behaviors, whereas *punishment* strategies aim to decrease undesirable behaviors. For example, telling a child that you noticed that they changed into their pajamas without reminders is rewarding a desired behavior, making it more likely that they do the same thing again the next night (with the hopes of getting positive attention for it again). A punishment strategy would involve taking away their electronic device because they did not change into their pajamas when directed to do so. Research shows that *punishment* strategies are not nearly as effective as positive reinforcement strategies in warding off undesirable behaviors. (Yep, you read that right—punishing bad behaviors is less effective than rewarding good ones!)

WAIT A MINUTE, ISN'T THAT BRIBERY?

Positively reinforcing desired behavior should not be confused with bribing children to follow expectations. Bribes are generally considered coercive. When a parent bribes a child, the reward (the bribe) is issued *before* the desired behavior. Positive behavioral rewards are issued *after* a desired behavior has taken place. For example, giving your child $20 as enticement to sleep in their own bed all night is a bribe; whereas preparing your child's favorite breakfast after they've slept in their own bed all night is a reward. We discourage the use of bribery in favor of positive reinforcement because the child who has been bribed (1) has missed out on an opportunity to freely choose to take on a challenge, earn the reward, and feel good about it, (2) fails to learn that rewards come from our efforts, (3) may learn to refuse parental requests unless the reward is provided up front (e.g., "I'll do it if you pay me first"), and, perhaps worst of all, (4) is not guaranteed to complete the task once the bribe has been issued!

Remember, parents may occasionally engage in behaviors that are consistent with more than one parenting style. No one particular behavior consistent with any of the parenting styles is necessarily bad—there may be times when a No Nonsense stance is necessary (e.g., child is dangerously close to a balcony edge), or when Anything Goes parenting is warranted (e.g., child is choosing their own clothing at a store). Nevertheless, one's parenting should, overall, align with the Balanced parenting style to promote good behavior and maximize child health, safety, and well-being. See table 2.1 to compare the warmth and firmness levels of the four parenting styles. Find out your parenting style with our Parenting Style Tracker. You can access it at the end of this week's reading. See figure 2.1 to see a completed Parenting Style Tracker.

FINDING THE BALANCE

Parents' accommodating behaviors tend to show up in response to a child's report of being uncomfortable or scared, and parents want to help them feel more at ease. We get that. But don't forget that accommodation has its drawbacks. It can send a subtle message that bedtime is, in fact, scary and that your child can't handle it on their own. It's quite common for children who don't sleep independently to feel somewhat uneasy or apprehensive at bedtime. Keep in mind that your child may describe the bedtime situation as "hard" or something they "just don't like" when what they are really feeling is uncomfortable or anxious. The good news is that a little bit of discomfort or nervousness at bedtime is normal! The even better news is that you have the power to help your

Table 2.1. The Four Parenting Styles

	Low Warmth	High Warmth
Low Firmness	You're On Your Own	Anything Goes
High Firmness	No Nonsense	Balanced

HIGH PERFORMANCE PARENTING
CHAMPION THEIR FUTURE

Parenting Style Tracker

At the end of each day, indicate the parenting behaviors you engaged in. Always strive for Balanced parenting behaviors.

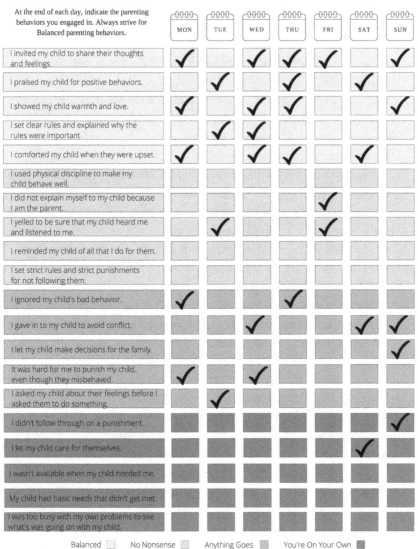

	MON	TUE	WED	THU	FRI	SAT	SUN
I invited my child to share their thoughts and feelings.	✓		✓	✓	✓		✓
I praised my child for positive behaviors.		✓		✓		✓	
I showed my child warmth and love.	✓		✓	✓			✓
I set clear rules and explained why the rules were important		✓	✓				
I comforted my child when they were upset.	✓		✓	✓		✓	
I used physical discipline to make my child behave well.							
I did not explain myself to my child because I am the parent.				✓			
I yelled to be sure that my child heard me and listened to me.		✓			✓		
I reminded my child of all that I do for them.							
I set strict rules and strict punishments for not following them.							
I ignored my child's bad behavior.	✓			✓			
I gave in to my child to avoid conflict.			✓			✓	✓
I let my child make decisions for the family.							✓
It was hard for me to punish my child, even though they misbehaved.	✓		✓				
I asked my child about their feelings before I asked them to do something.		✓					
I didn't follow through on a punishment.							✓
I let my child care for themselves.						✓	
I wasn't available when my child needed me.							
My child had basic needs that didn't get met.							
I was too busy with my own problems to see what's was going on with my child.							

Balanced   No Nonsense   Anything Goes   You're On Your Own

Figure 2.1. Sample Parenting Style Tracker. *Source:* High Performance Parenting (www.highperformance-parenting.com)

child face the bedtime challenge by responding in an intentional and . . . you guessed it . . . warm and firm way.

Table 2.2 presents common, but unhelpful, accommodations that parents tend to make for their child at bedtime, as well as how to go about "undoing" these accommodations (i.e., promoting independence in your child). The table is designed to illustrate the differences between Anything Goes parenting and Balanced parenting and is not intended to present quick fixes. Modifying parental behavior to recognize and remove unhelpful accommodations will require your time and attention. If some of the accommodations presented below are relevant to your child, be mindful that they won't automatically know how to cope with the distress that some of these newly independent activities may bring on. Weeks 3–6 will provide you with detailed instruction on how to support your child's coping.

You and your parenting partner may have different parenting styles. Many times, it's advantageous as one parent can serve to even out the other. We've often worked with couples where one parent is "warm" and the other is "firm." Though this can set the stage for a lot of conflict, it can also be the foundation for warm and firm parenting! If the parents work together, meeting in the middle, they will likely find the parenting sweet spot.

Sometimes that sweet spot can be elusive. If you and your parenting co-partner have a contentious relationship, this could make your child more likely to experience sleep difficulties. Less-than-ideal co-parenting, family or partner conflict, and parental anxiety and depression have been found to be risk factors for child sleep problems.[2] We know it's not always possible to sidestep conflict in the midst of real-life stressors including job pressures, financial worries, family emergencies, and other life events demanding your attention and taking a toll on your mental health. Who can think about sleep when the proverbial house is on fire? If your homelife isn't as tranquil as you'd like, you might consider taking steps to improve not only your co-parenting, but

Table 2.2. Anything Goes and Balanced Parenting Behaviors for Common Bedtime Accommodations

Anything Goes Parenting Behaviors (With bedtime accommodations) If you currently . . .	Balanced Parenting Behaviors (Without bedtime accommodations) Do this instead . . .
Place water and snacks on your child's nightstand before bed to avoid nighttime complaints of thirst and hunger.	Explain to your child that there is no eating after bedtime. Ensure that your child eats and drinks *before* getting into bed (see table 1.2 for recommended foods before bed).
Turn off your child's bedroom light once your child has been tucked in because they are unwilling to get out of their bed in the dark.	Have your child turn off their own bedroom light as a signal they are ready to be "tucked in."
Let your two children share a bedroom due to one's fear of being alone at night.	Invite the siblings to earn a special weekend activity to celebrate independent sleep successes and help them maintain a close bond.
Do a "sweep" of your child's closet before bedtime because they are afraid of monsters dwelling there.	Tell your child that you are *so* confident that there are no monsters in their closet that you don't even have to check (and refrain from checking it!).
Walk ahead of your child to their bedroom because they're uncomfortable leading the way.	Walk with your child by your side. Once they get used to that (it may take days), have them walk just ahead of you, perhaps one step at a time.
Promise your child that you'll remain nearby as they go to sleep.	Tell your child that you'll be "around," and you are confident that they can go to sleep on their own.

Anything Goes Parenting Behaviors (With bedtime accommodations) If you currently . . .	Balanced Parenting Behaviors (Without bedtime accommodations) Do this instead . . .
Give in to your child's demands for a later bedtime (for any number of reasons—you are tired, your child is relentless, siblings will wake up if the child cries or tantrums).	Explain to your child, "I understand that you want to stay up later. I used to feel like that when I was your age too (warm), but it's my job to make sure that you get enough sleep, so I'm holding firm to your bedtime (firm)."
Put a TV in your child's room because they say all their friends have TVs.	Talk with your child about what makes sleep difficult for kids. "I totally get it. I love to watch TV at night too (warm), but when we do, it negatively affects our sleep so I will not allow it (firm)."
Proceed with Caution If you currently . . .	Be advised . . .
Let your child sleep on the living room couch instead of in their bedroom.	Children's bedtime preferences may or may not be related to fear or anxiety. If your child can be flexible (e.g., some nights sleeping on the living room couch and other nights not), odds are that the behavior is a preference and not an anxious behavior so go ahead and allow it. But if your child is inflexible (e.g., refuses to sleep anywhere but on the couch), there is a good chance that your child is anxious about sleeping alone in their bedroom. Then, you'll want to use warm and firm parenting to eliminate the accommodation (e.g., gradually move your child to a sleeping location closer and closer to their own bedroom).

also the relationship with your co-parent and your mental health through individual or couples counseling, or family therapy. When you take time to improve relationships and reduce conflicts, your child learns important lessons in persistence, managing conflict, the value of doing hard work, and remaining hopeful for the future—and, odds are, everyone's sleep will improve.

Balanced parenting will go a long way toward building your child's cooperation, compliance, and self-confidence. We've got additional tools in the toolbox, though, to enhance your child's competence and ability to cope in a wide range of difficult situations. Ahead, you'll find vignettes that will demonstrate how to put plans into action. In Week 3, you'll help your child master some fundamental skills needed for navigating difficult bedtime (and daytime) situations. These skills will help your child enjoy better sleep, less stress, and lower anxiety. They can also use these skills to persist longer in difficult tasks, better navigate difficult situations, keep their calm when they need it most, and develop a belief in their own ability to handle demanding situations. Read on to give your child's coping skills a boost in Week 3. Week 3 will also guide you in beginning to alter your child's sleeping environment to provide conditions that will maximize good sleep.

 Now Apply It!

Become more aware of your parenting practices. Over the next week, complete the Parenting Style Tracker worksheet.* Self-monitoring will help you to examine the link between your parenting behaviors and their effect on your child's moods, behaviors, and self-esteem, as well as on the home environment more generally.

*Access the worksheet by scanning the QR code below or by going to www.highperformance-parenting.com/bbb -appendices.

Week 2 Summary

- A parenting style is the way that a parent parents. It's important to understand one's parenting style because it directly impacts child outcomes, including bedtime behaviors and, therefore, sleep.

- One's parenting style tends to fall within one of four main categories: No Nonsense, You're On Your Own, Anything Goes, and Balanced.

- No Nonsense parenting involves extremely strict rules without child input or compromise and tends to result in child emotional and behavioral issues. If the parenting is exceedingly harsh or severe, this style of parenting can be considered abusive.

- You're On Your Own parenting, leaving the child to their own devices often to a neglectful degree, may result in child emotional and behavioral problems.

- Anything Goes parenting involves often "giving in" to the child's demands. This also involves accommodating the child's fears, which reduces anxiety in the short-term, but maintains or even strengthens anxiety in the long-term. Parents of children with persistent nighttime fears, for example, may have permissive parenting tendencies around the child's bedtime routine. Anything Goes parenting also sets the stage for child emotional and behavioral difficulties.

- Balanced parenting involves empathy, structure, positive reinforcement, and boundaries (we call this being "warm and firm"). This style is best in most circumstances because it supports the child's emotional well-being and is most effective for accomplishing desired behavioral outcomes, such as independent sleeping. In the upcoming weeks, you will learn how to apply Balanced parenting strategies at bedtime to help your child become an independent sleeper.

WEEK 3

Build Your Child's Coping Skills

THIS WEEK YOU WILL TACKLE THREE IMPORTANT TASKS: (1) building your child's calming and coping skills, (2) helping your child to develop a sleep-promoting mindset, and (3) creating a sleep-promoting environment in your child's bedroom. We'll walk you through each of these tasks to ensure that your changes are on the right track and sustainable for the long-term.

HELP YOUR CHILD LEARN TO RELAX

First, you will start building your child's skills to manage the inevitable discomfort that will initially come with sleeping independently. You will learn about two important coping skills to assist in calming their body and mind: (1) mindful deep breathing and (2) progressive muscle relaxation.

In our experience, many, though not all, children take to these skills right away. Many find the exercises to be essential tools in their coping tool kit. If your child voices opposition to learning the skills, encourage them to give the exercises a chance. Like any skill to be learned, it takes practice before your child can reap the benefits!

Mindful Breathing

Mindfulness, very simply, is the act of being *aware* of what is happening in the present moment. Being mindful is more than what it seems. This is because humans are often thinking about past events (even those that happened only moments ago) in an effort to avoid repeating mistakes and about possible future events in an effort to prevent bad things from happening. Though there is value in considering the past and planning for the future, we often don't spend enough time fully aware of what is happening in the present, which is where life is happening! Plus, one is less likely to feel depressed (past-focused) or anxious (future-focused) when the focus is kept squarely on the here and now.

Want to try some mindfulness? Start with your senses. Notice a sound in your environment. How loud is it? Is it steady or intermittent? From where is the sound emanating? Close or far away? Next, try being mindful of where your body meets your seat. Notice the degree of cushion. How long can you focus on that sensation? Chances are good that your thoughts quickly began to jump around. We never said practicing mindfulness was easy. It takes a lot of practice to be able to maintain focus on the present moment, but it's worth the effort! Mindfulness may be especially important in mitigating the negative effects on mental health brought on by the COVID-19 pandemic. A recent study found that mindfulness protects people from psychological distress brought on by the pandemic.[1]

Mindful breathing requires a focus on one's breathing. Take a few deep breaths and notice how your body feels when you inhale and how it feels when you exhale. Breathing slowly and deeply facilitates the body's natural relaxation response. Deep breathing corrects the rapid and shallow breathing that often occurs during periods of distress. Rapid shallow breathing can lead to hyperventilation, dizziness, and lightheadedness. Taking deep, full breaths, on the other hand, produces feelings of calm and relaxation. Go ahead. Try it! Slowing down one's breathing not only promotes feelings of relaxation, but it also improves body functioning and calms the mind, making sleep much easier to achieve.

Teach your child to use mindful deep breathing using the steps below. You'll begin the mindful deep breathing exercise *with* your child, but eventually, you'll want your child to do the mindful deep breathing exercise on their own. A useful strategy for promoting the skill in your child is "see one, do one, teach one": illustrate proper breathing to your child first ("see one"), before having them try it on their own ("do one"). At this stage, your child may prefer to use a guided audio or video to breathe along with. Then, once your child can reliably follow the proper breathing technique independently, have them teach it back to you or to a relative or friend ("teach one")! To teach mindful deep breathing, read the *italic* words in the four steps below to your child. The following mindful deep breathing script takes approximately four to five minutes to read aloud.

Scripted Steps to Teach Your Child Mindful Deep Breathing

Step #1: *Deep breathing is a powerful tool for relaxing your body and mind. You can use it anytime you want to take a break or when you're feeling especially worried or overwhelmed. It's especially good to use at night while you are lying in bed ready to go to sleep.*

Step #2: *Put one hand on your stomach and the other hand on your chest. Pay attention to your breathing. Which hand is doing more of the moving?*

(If the hand on the chest is moving and the hand on the stomach is still, this is not deep breathing. Have them work toward switching this around—so the hand on the stomach rises and falls more so than the hand on the chest.)

Take slow, deep breaths and try to make the hand on your stomach move and keep your hand on your chest as still as possible. The hand on your stomach should go up as you breathe in and down as you breathe out.

Step #3: *Keep taking deep, steady breaths. Try breathing in through your nose and out through your mouth.* Inhales and exhales should each last a few seconds.

Note: If your child has a lung or heart condition, they might have difficulty with deep breathing. If they report difficulty, slow the process down and help them to complete the exercise comfortably.

Step #4: *Let's practice this exercise every day so we can get really good at relaxing our body through breathing. One of the great things about this strategy is that you can use it anywhere without anyone noticing! Can you think of some situations when this type of breathing would be helpful?*

Tips for mindful deep breathing: (1) Have your child purse their lips (as if blowing through a straw) while exhaling as this will help them control the flow of their exhale, (2) Have your child close their eyes during the practice to prevent distractions and deepen the relaxation response, and (3) Suggest your child use a mantra such as "calm" or "relax" during each exhale.

Progressive Muscle Relaxation (PMR)

Relaxation techniques are designed to reduce tension, stress, worry, and anxiety. Progressive Muscle Relaxation (PMR) is a type of relaxation that consists of tensing and then relaxing various muscle groups throughout the body. Using PMR, your child will learn how to recognize tension in their body and then relax the tense muscles, which feels calming and prevents additional distress (muscle aches, headaches, tantrums, etc.).

When introducing PMR to your child, be sure your child understands the reasons for using PMR and why it may be good for them. You can explain PMR in the following way: *When we get stressed out, upset, or worried, our bodies naturally tighten up our muscles like this* (demonstrate tight muscles to your child by balling up your fist). *We might not even notice that we are doing it! This can leave us feeling pretty tired at the end of the day. Tensing muscles all day is a bit like doing exercise but without all the benefits. When we learn to notice tense muscles and then relax them, our body feels more comfortable, and our minds can think more easily and clearly.*

Next, show them how it's done. Following the "see one, do one, teach one" method, have your child master the skill independently before teaching the strategy to someone else. Instructions for this exercise are below (read the *italic* words in the five steps below to your child).

Steps to Teach Your Child Progressive Muscle Relaxation (PMR)

Step #1: Learn PMR to make it easier to feel relaxed. *I'm going to teach you how to tell the difference between feeling tense and feeling relaxed, and how to create a feeling of relaxation. It feels good when we are relaxed.* (Make sure that your child understands what "tense" means. You can illustrate this by flexing your muscles and contrasting that tension with a loose, nonflexed muscle.)

Step #2: Note the difference between the feelings of tension and relaxation. *Whenever we feel tense, we can help our body relax. But we've got to practice this to get good at it. When we're stressed, our muscles can gradually become more tense without us realizing it. The good news is that you can stop and loosen them up using what I'm about to teach you—something called progressive muscle relaxation.*

Step #3: Tense and relax different muscle groups. *Progressive muscle relaxation is when you tense and relax different muscle groups one at a time, starting with your hands and arms, then shoulders, face, neck, stomach, legs, and feet. When tensing each specific muscle group, tense only that muscle group (not ALL of your muscles at the same time—that would be too uncomfortable!). While we practice this skill, concentrate on how your body feels.* Ask your child to describe bodily sensations—*How does your body feel right now? What are you noticing?* Help your child notice the way their body "feels" when tense versus when relaxed. See the time-honored PMR script below[2] (some elements are modified for present-day use).

Step #4: Discuss your child's experiences. After the relaxation exercise, ask your child their thoughts about the muscle relaxation practice—*How does your body feel now? What was that like for you?*

Modify the procedures if your child experienced any pain while tensing their muscles. Tensing should not be painful.

Step #5: Encourage regular practice. Help your child practice PMR at least once a day to develop mastery over the technique and help them recognize its benefits. Like any skill, PMR takes practice, so don't let your child give up too soon. It may take a few weeks for the skill to achieve maximum benefits. As your child becomes more experienced with PMR, they may be able to skip the tensing part and go straight to relaxing the various muscle groups. PMR is great to practice at night in bed. Make it part of the bedtime routine!

Progressive Muscle Relaxation (PMR) Practice Sessions

To begin a relaxation session, have your child sit comfortably in a chair and close their eyes. Relaxing music or calming white noise such as sounds of rain or waves may be played in the background. When reading the script, speak in a soft, even tone. Read more slowly than is typical for you. Alternatively, you can find numerous audio and video versions of this PMR script with a quick online search.

Hands and Arms. *Pretend you have a lemon in your left hand. Now squeeze it to try to get all the juice out. Feel the tightness in your hand and arm as you squeeze. Now drop the lemon. Notice how your muscles feel when they are relaxed. Take another lemon and squeeze it. Try to squeeze it harder than you did the first one. That's right. Real hard. Now drop your lemon and relax. Notice how much better your hand and arm feel when they are relaxed. Once again, take a lemon in your left hand and try to squeeze all the juice out. Don't leave a single drop. Squeeze hard. Now relax and let the lemon fall from your hand.* (Repeat this process with the right hand and arm.)

Arms and Shoulders. *Pretend you are a furry, lazy cat. You want to stretch. Stretch your arms out in front of you. Place them up high over your head, way back. Feel the pull in your shoulders. Stretch higher. Now just let your arms drop back to your side. Okay, let's stretch again. Stretch your arms out in front of you. Raise them over your head. Put them back, way back. Pull hard. Now let them drop quickly. This time let's have a great big stretch. Try to touch the ceiling. Stretch your arms way out in front of you. Raise them way up high over your head. Push them way, way back. Notice the tension and pull in your arms and shoulders. Hold tight now. Great. Let them drop quickly and feel how good it is to be relaxed. It feels good and warm and lazy.*

Shoulders and Neck. *Now pretend you are a turtle. You're sitting on a rock by a lake or a peaceful pond just relaxing in the warm sun. It feels nice and warm and safe here. Uh-oh! You sense danger. Pull your head into your shell. Try to pull your shoulders up to your ears and push your head down into your shoulders. Hold in tight. It isn't easy to be a turtle in a shell. The danger is past now. You can come out into the warm sunshine and once again relax. Watch out now! More danger. Hurry, pull your head back into your shell and hold it tight. You must be closed in tight to protect yourself. Okay, you can relax now. Raise your head out of your shell and let your shoulders relax. Notice how much better it feels to be relaxed than to be all tight. One more time now! Danger! Pull your head in. Push your shoulders way up to your ears and hold tight. Don't let even a tiny piece of your head show outside your shell. Hold it. Feel the tenseness in your neck and shoulders. You can come out now. It's safe again. Relax and feel comfortable. There's no danger. Nothing to worry about. Nothing to be afraid of. You feel good.*

Jaw. *You have a giant piece of bubble gum in your mouth. It's very hard to chew. Bite down on it. Hard! Let your neck muscles help you. Now relax. Just let your jaw hang loose. Notice how good it feels just to let your jaw drop. Okay, let's tackle that bubble gum again. Bite down. Hard! Try to squeeze it out between your teeth. That's good. You're really tearing that gum up. Now relax again. Just let your jaw drop off your face. It feels so good just to let go and not have to fight that bubble gum. Okay, one more time. We're really going to tear it up this time. Bite down. Hard as you can. Harder. Oh, you're really working hard. Good. Now relax. Try to relax your whole body. You've beaten the bubble gum. Let yourself go as loose as you can.*

Stomach. *This time imagine that you are playing soccer with a friend. Suddenly, your friend kicks the ball hard and it's headed directly for your stomach. Knowing you can't use your hands in soccer, you tighten your stomach muscles to get ready for the impact. Brace for the hit. Try to get your belly button to touch your backbone. Good! Now relax your stomach muscles. The ball bounced far away, and you can let your stomach relax. Okay, instant replay! It's happening again. Tighten up your stomach. Get it real tight. Hold it. Instant replay complete. You can relax now. Settle back and let your stomach feel loose and warm. You can feel really good now. You're doing great.*

Legs and Feet. *Now pretend that you are standing barefoot in a big, fat mud puddle. Squish your toes down deep into the mud. Try to get your feet down to the bottom of the mud puddle. You'll probably need your legs to help you push. Push down, spread your toes apart, and feel the mud squish up between your toes. Now step out of the mud puddle. Relax your feet. Let your toes go loose and feel how nice that is. It feels good to be relaxed. Go back into the mud puddle. Squish your toes down. Let your leg muscles help push your feet down. Push your feet. Hard. Try to squeeze that mud puddle dry. Okay, come back out now. Relax your feet, relax your legs, relax your toes. It feels so good to be relaxed. No tenseness anywhere. You feel warm and tingly.*

Now, stay as relaxed as you can. Let your whole body go limp and feel all your muscles relaxed. In a few minutes I will ask you to open your eyes, and that will be the end of this session. Afterward, remember how good it feels to be relaxed. Sometimes you have to make yourself more tense before you can be relaxed, just as we did in these exercises. Practice these exercises every day to get more and more relaxed. A good time to practice is at night, after you have gone to bed and the lights are out and you won't be disturbed. It will help you fall asleep. Then, when you are a really good relaxer, you can help yourself relax at home, school, or anywhere. Just remember the turtle, or the bubble gum, or the mud puddle, and you can do these exercises and nobody will know.

You've worked hard today, and it feels good to work hard. Very slowly, now, open your eyes and wiggle your muscles around a little. Very good. You've done a good job. You're going to be a super relaxer.

CREATE A SLEEP-PROMOTING MINDSET

How does your child perceive bedtime? You can probably make a reasonable guess based on what they tell you and how they behave at bedtime. A positive perception of bedtime is crucial if you want to banish the bedtime battles once and for all. If bedtime doesn't currently call to mind fluffy pillows and snuggly blankets for your child, not all hope is lost. We can help. To foster a sleep-promoting mindset, you'll first need to understand the relationships among thoughts, emotions, and actions.

To start, let's consider a situation—any situation at all. For illustration purposes, let's think back to this morning when your child was eating their breakfast. At that time, your child had a thought about breakfast: "Mom made my *favorite* breakfast." Then their thought generated an emotion or feeling (cheerful and satisfied). That emotional state then motivated action (your child chats happily about their day).

To recap:

Situation: Your child is eating their favorite breakfast.

Child's Thought: *Mom made my* favorite *breakfast.*

Child's Emotion: Cheerful and satisfied.

Child's Action: Chats happily with you about their day.

Let's take another example—one that may be a bit more typical:

Situation: Your child is playing on their iPad, and you tell them it's time to get ready for bed.

Child's Thought: *But I want to keep playing!*

Child's Emotion: Frustrated.

Child's Action: Ignores you and keeps playing.

Sounds familiar, right? Now, let's imagine that we want to end up with a different outcome (who wouldn't in this situation?). We want the child to respond quickly to our request to get ready for bed and with a pleasant demeanor. So let's try an intervention: using this same situation, let's substitute the thought, "*But I want to keep playing!*" with a new and different thought.

(Same) Situation: Your child is playing on their iPad, and you tell them it's time to get ready for bed.

Child's Thought: *It's time for bed.*

Child's Emotion: Calm.

Child's Action: Transitions off the iPad and gets ready for bed.

You can see how altering a single thought can lead to a different outcome. In other words, if you don't like how you're feeling or behaving, trace that feeling and behavior back to a thought and then exchange it for something else that's more helpful. In the psychology world, changing a thought, or set of thoughts, is known as "cognitive restructuring" and is well-known for helping with emotion regulation and behavior change.

You might be wondering how you can plug a thought of your choice into your child's head so you can get the outcome you're looking for. You can't. Well, not directly. But we do have a way to prime the pump, so to speak. Let's imagine that your child has trouble quieting their mind at night. They are wrapped up in their worries about things that happened during the day and already anticipating the things that might go wrong tomorrow. You want them to think about something else—to think a bit differently. Sounds like a time for cognitive restructuring!

Gently determine what it is that your child is worried about (determine the situation and their thoughts). We've got the emotion in the bag—we know that they are feeling anxious and worried. Next, use the following strategy to prompt a change in your child's thinking. Ask, "What's another way to think about this situation?" or "What might you say to a friend or a sibling who was in this same situation?" Encouraging your child to take on different perspectives teaches them a critical life skill. They'll see that they can begin to think and feel differently about a situation, even when (*especially* when) they cannot change the situation! Wow, that's powerful.

Let's see that superpower in action:

Situation: Sarina is cuddling with her mother at bedtime on a school night.

Sarina's Thought: *I won't be able to fall asleep by myself.*

Sarina's Emotion: Worried.

Sarina's Action: Pleads with her mother to lay with her until she falls asleep.

Sarina's mother asks her, "What are some other ways to think about this situation?"

Sarina and her mother brainstorm a few alternative thoughts and Sarina selects one that she feels might be helpful.

Sarina's New Thoughts: *My body knows what to do. I've slept thousands of hours on my own. Besides, even if I'm tired tomorrow, it won't be the worst thing in the world.*

Sarina's New Emotion: Self-assured.

Sarina's New Action: She gives sleeping on her own a try.

So we can't conduct a thought-ectomy, where we remove and replace a child's thoughts, but we can indirectly influence their thoughts and perceptions of situations, including bedtime. We want your child to begin to think differently about what it means to go to bed. We want them to shift from hating the thought of bedtime to appreciating the end of the day and the restorative power of sleep. We've already demonstrated one method of influence, but we've got another up our sleeve! If you want a major boost in your child's ability to think differently about bedtime and sleep, model positive family attitudes toward bedtime and sleep.

If you change how *you* think and talk about sleep, you can alter your child's thinking about sleep. Many adults, parents included, often express a love-hate relationship with sleep. In any given exchange, you might hear another adult say, "I get no sleep these days; hopefully I can sleep tonight," "I'll sleep when I'm dead," or "Is it time to go to bed already?!" These folks are essentially communicating that sleep is elusive, irrelevant, a waste of time, or something to be dreaded. If you feel this way, and as a result speak about sleep this way in front of your child, they will likely learn to adopt this mindset too, which could contribute to the bedtime problems you're experiencing.

Even if you haven't openly disparaged sleep in front of your child, chances are that your verbal and nonverbal messaging around sleep could use a boost. See table 3.1 below for some dos and don'ts when it comes to talking about sleep.

CREATE A SLEEP-PROMOTING ENVIRONMENT

You'll recall that we discussed important features of an optimal bedtime sleeping environment in Week 1. To review, factors that interfere with falling and staying asleep include technology use, light, and noise. In general, the aim is to reduce distractions and ensure a quiet and restful sleeping environment. Now's not the time to change elements that are likely to cause your child some distress (e.g., removing a night-light). This week, you are going to get a head start on enhancing the sleep environment by changing elements that your child is unlikely to notice.

To start, ensure that your child's bedroom is cool (less than 72 degrees if possible). If you live in a region where it can get very cold during the nights, be sure that your child has blankets for warmth. If your climate is a hot one, invest in a small fan for the bedroom. Next, do the best you can to ensure a quiet sleeping environment. This could involve asking family members to restrict any noisy activities to earlier in the day (this will likely help them sleep better as well!). You might make a family policy of quiet activity after 7 or 8 p.m. If sounds of talking, laughing, or TV drift into your child's bedroom, consider whether it is reasonable or feasible to switch rooms. For example, can loud conversations

Table 3.1. Positively Influence Your Child's Perception of Sleep

DO	DON'T
Verbal Messaging	
Talk to your child about the nourishing benefits of sleep for their brain and body.	Tell your child that they have to go to bed "because I said so."
Say, about your own sleep, "I *want to* go to sleep at 9 p.m. so that my brain and body are at their best tomorrow."	Say, "I should have gone to sleep hours ago."
Normalize the balance of daytime excitement and bedtime wind down. Say something like, "Our family is busy by day and tranquil by night."	Refer to bedtime as "boring."
Say, "My favorite part of the day is spending quiet time with you at bedtime."	Tell your child they need to go to bed so you can have a break from them.
Tell your child how good it feels to go to bed feeling so safe and cozy.	Warn your child about bed bugs or monsters under the bed.

DO	DON'T
Nonverbal Messaging	
Find at least one way to enjoy the evening in a family space (e.g., put on easy listening music, light a candle, build a "slow" evening activity into your routine such as reading, doing a crossword puzzle, journaling, or savoring a cup of tea).	Skip engaging in adult wind-down activities or doing so only out of your children's sight.
Create positive bedtime associations.	Tell your child to go to bed as a punishment for demonstrating unwanted behavior.
Keep your own bedroom as tidy and inviting for *your* sleep as possible.	Use your bedroom primarily as the family's laundry sorting station.
Store electronic devices outside of your bedroom.	Routinely use your phone while in bed.
Use a warm tone when talking about sleep and bedtime directives.	Raise your voice at bedtime due to fatigue and frustration with your child's behavior.

move into a room farther from your child's bedroom or can the child's bedroom be swapped to a location in the home that is a bit quieter? These changes may be inconvenient, but be sure to take a long-range view—while it is a pain to move furniture around, will the result mean years of improved sleep for everyone in the home? If so, the trouble is likely worth it.

Next, help your child forge a strong connection between sleep and their bed. Principles of learning tell us that if two things are repeatedly paired over time, such as your child's bed and sleep, they develop a strong association. So when your child crawls into bed, sleep should come rather quickly due to the strong association. Many parents use products in the sleeping environment which can, through the association with sleep, make sleep easier to come by. Products that are scented (e.g., lotions, sprays) or have a comforting touch (e.g., soft or weighted blanket) or sound (e.g., wind chimes outside the window, sound machines, low frequency music/binaural beats) can all become associated with the onset of sleep.

While these associations can be very powerful in facilitating sleep, beware of the possibility of developing an overreliance on them. For example, what if you run out of the lavender pillow spray, or worse yet, the product is discontinued? What if the spray is forgotten at home when your family travels? What happens if your child is invited to sleep at a friend's home? Some temporary use of these items can be helpful in the transition to independent sleeping, but recognize that these aids should be used on a relatively short-term basis and phased out before too long.

Above, we talked about creating positive sleep associations in which something becomes paired with sleep and thus helps your child fall asleep. Due to the relative ease of creating sleep associations, however, this process can work against you as well. Consider what might happen if your child uses their bed for a variety of activities, including studying, using screens, or eating. Due to the power of sleep associations, these activities can serve to weaken the association we are striving to build (i.e., bed–sleep) and strengthen associations that make falling asleep more difficult (e.g., bed–studying, bed–screen use, and bed–eating). So your child's bed should be off-limits except for sleeping. To help in this, you may want to get rid of any accessories (e.g., bed rest pillows, bed trays) that help one engage in non-sleep activities while in bed.

Your child's bedroom should be free of stimulating elements. For some of you, this is not so simple because some children have stimulating elements paired with their sleep onset such as watching YouTube videos on an iPad until they fall asleep. It's unlikely that your child will be able to give up this stimulating element easily; so, for this week, focus on those elements that will be easier to eliminate, such as reducing natural light in the bedroom through use of curtains, shades, or other light-blocking options. In a couple of weeks, you'll work on removing other elements which are likely to provoke strong complaints from your child, such as night-lights and electronic devices.

It is likely (and desirable) that your skill practice (mindful deep breathing, progressive muscle relaxation) takes place in your child's bedroom. This is good—it will help your child to pair the relaxation response with the physical location of their bedroom. Some children require additional efforts to feel comfortable in their bedroom. If this is your child, have them begin to spend some time alone (e.g., playing, reading, listening to music) in their bedroom during the morning and early afternoon hours. Then gradually have them progress toward spending time alone in their room in the late afternoons and early evenings. This will help them adjust to being alone in their bedroom in the evening and throughout the night. They'll gradually become comfortable being alone in their bedroom, and you'll enjoy a few child-free moments as well.

It is also helpful to use visual and auditory reminders of coping strategies and incentives (rewards) that may be part of your child's sleep plan. Help your child decorate their room with reminders of their ability to cope with everyday stress. You can use inspirational quotes, supportive notes, pictures, or audio reminders (e.g., voice-controlled virtual assistants such as Alexa, set to announce coping statements or encouragement, calming music), as well as other sensory input (e.g., fish tank, choice of bedroom paint colors, tapestry). Get your child in on the action! Their help with the creation of these supports will increase both their motivation and commitment to the upcoming sleep plan.

 Now Apply It!

1. Teach your child the coping skills introduced this week (mindful deep breathing and progressive muscle relaxation) and have them practice daily.

2. Encourage a sleep-promoting mindset in your child by prompting them to consider things from different vantage points when they are distressed at bedtime. Ask your child for other ways to look at the situation. Pose the following questions to your child:

   a. "What's another way to think about this situation?"

   b. "What might you say to a friend in the same situation?"

3. Be mindful of your attitude and communication about sleep in front of your child. Play up the benefits of a good night's sleep.

4. Modify your child's bedroom environment according to the recommendations outlined this week. Take some time to create and decorate with coping materials. Use some of our inspirational posters* or make your own.

5. Review the ideal bedtime routine that you created during Week 1. Tweak as needed before implementation in Week 5. Be sure that any parenting partners have had a chance to review, offer suggestions, and indicate their support of the plan. Next week, you'll have the opportunity to present this plan to your child. For now, refine the plan with suggestions from other caregivers.

*Access the posters by scanning the QR code below or by going to www.highperformance-parenting.com/bbb -appendices.

WEEK 3 SUMMARY

- Doing new things can be stressful for everyone, especially children. Your child will benefit from learning how to calm their mind and body so that they can tolerate distress brought on by new situations. Of course, a calm mind and body also set the stage for sleep.

- Mindful deep breathing and progressive muscle relaxation are two calming techniques that your child can learn relatively quickly and use as part of an independent bedtime routine.

- Create a sleep-promoting mindset by (1) helping your child discover alternate ways to think about worries and concerns, and (2) being mindful about how you think and talk about sleep.

- Create a sleep-promoting environment by cooling down the room, removing stimulation, and enhancing your child's sleep associations.

WEEK 4

Pick Your Battles

WELCOME TO WEEK 4, WHERE YOU'LL LEARN WHAT YOU AND your child need to do for them to sleep independently in their own bed . . . without the battles. There's much to look forward to! Now that you have in place the sleep basics, an effective parenting style, calming strategies, and a sleep-supportive environment from your efforts during previous weeks, you're ready for some high-quality parenting moves! Week 5 will be individualized based on the bedtime battle(s) you encounter most frequently, but first you need to know ten key parenting strategies on which you will rely during the implementation phase.

TEN PARENTING STRATEGIES FOR CHILD INDEPENDENT SLEEP AND BEYOND

No matter what bedtime battle(s) you are facing, you will be using some combination of the following ten strategies pertinent to the goal of independent sleep.

1. Provide Clear Communication and Structure

Like many things in life, a successful bedtime routine is rooted in good communication. For your child to experience a happy and healthy bedtime routine, you must identify your expectations for bedtime and the consequences of not following those expectations, communicate to your child exactly what you expect from them, *and* ensure that your child understands precisely what you mean. Communication of expectations should be verbal and visual (e.g., display a list of expectations somewhere in the home). Consequences for not following expectations may be "natural" (e.g., reading time is 8:30 p.m. to 8:45 p.m., so getting into bed past 8:30 p.m. cuts into reading time). Discuss the expectations and consequences with your child to check for their understanding of them.

Once you have provided clear communication about bedtime expectations, then ongoing communication, monitoring, and support are necessary. Structure is the next place to focus. The Apple Dictionary app defines *structure* as "the arrangement of and relations between the parts or elements of something complex." Bedtime is nothing if not complex! A structured bedtime consists of mutually agreed-upon behaviors carried out at a designated time, in a general order, with some-but-not-too-much parental support. So how do you create this structure? Once you have verbally communicated your expectations, you must continually communicate them on a regular basis. Ongoing communication of expectations contributes to a structured bedtime and can take the form of verbal, visual, and auditory cues aimed at promoting independence. Verbalize expectations (as needed) throughout the bedtime routine without emotionality (that means without obvious frustration, anger, disappointment, annoyance, or yelling). Expectations are nonnegotiable and, therefore, you should forgo the use of "please" and "thank you."

Visual and auditory cues or reminders can include positioning a clock in the living room as a silent reminder of the approaching bedtime, or if you own a voice-controlled virtual assistive device, such as Alexa or Google Home, it might be set to announce reminders of the approaching bedtime—these reminders can be humorous! Imagine Alexa announcing, "Now is the hour that all individuals under five feet begin nighttime preparations for slumber." (Parental monitoring is still important if you go the Alexa route.) The use of a structured bedtime supports the development of routine habits and practices that will last a lifetime. Keep reading to learn how to maintain this structure when your child protests the new bedtime routine.

2. Ritualize Parent-Child Togetherness

Rituals streamline our lives. Morning routines, taking the same path through your grocery store, and family traditions bring us comfort and stability. Rituals with your child are important because they provide them with comfort, security, and a sense of control, all of which are essential during times of stress.

The ritual of one-on-one time between parent and child at bedtime offers numerous benefits. Research with infants has demonstrated how important physical touch is to child health and development.[1] But don't limit your physical contact to infancy! Use positive physical contact (back rub, hand-holding, hug, fist bump) as your child grows. Research suggests that parent-child contact enhances health outcomes and well-being beyond infancy and across one's lifespan.[2] Parent interactions and subsequent child learning outcomes are negatively impacted by technology use, so technology-free time together is best. Prioritize quality time together at bedtime, but not for too long; keep it between five to fifteen minutes. If this isn't enough time together, add more time *before* the start of the bedtime routine.

3. Support Your Child's Use of Self-Regulation Strategies

Your child is learning how to regulate, or manage, their emotions. This is a developmental process that can be enhanced with your guidance. At bedtime, it is common for children to experience anxiety about monsters, noises, shadows, and so on. If your child becomes anxious about the prospect of sleeping independently, their body will gear up in anticipation. Their fight-or-flight system (the system of the body that reacts when we perceive danger—real or imagined) will respond by increasing heart rate, releasing adrenalin, constricting blood vessels—all of which make sleeping near impossible! When the body is responding to a perceived danger, sleeping would be foolhardy (think of whether you want to sleep if you encounter a bear while camping in the woods).

To set the stage for sleep to occur, your child must engage in behaviors that "turn off" the fight-or-flight response. This is where coping skills come in. Coping skills, specifically the calming kind, will help to quiet and calm your child's body and mind, paving the way for sleep. Achieve this with the mindful deep breathing, progressive muscle relaxation coping strategies, and sleep-promoting mindset from Week 3.

4. Use Shaping to Achieve Desired Behavior

We can influence others' behavior by rewarding specific behaviors that get closer and closer to the behavior we are hoping to see. For example, you shaped your child's behaviors when they learned to walk. You once encouraged your child to pull themselves up on all fours in preparation for a crawl. Then you stopped cheering on that behavior in favor of cheering on actual forward movement. Once your child mastered crawling, you again stopped rewarding crawling and instead cheered on standing, then those precious first steps, then walking! This is shaping—we reward closer and closer approximations to the desired behavior (walking, in this example).

This shaping procedure will be very helpful in getting your child to sleep independently. The kind of shaping needed depends on your child's current difficulties. If your child is fearful of going to sleep without you present, then one goal would be to gradually increase the physical distance between you and your child at bedtime. If your child wants every light in the home illuminated at night, then the goal would be to gradually reduce the number of lights or the brightness of lights. Shaping can also be used to reduce reliance on a fan or other sound for sleep. *All* parents will need to use the shaping technique, in one form or another, to move from your child's current bedtime routine to the desired bedtime routine. Shaping can be a parent's best friend when it is done gradually, consistently, and according to a plan. We'll return to this topic in Week 5. Stay tuned!

5. Limit the Number and Length of Interactions between You and Your Child Post-Bedtime

It is tempting to respond to your child's attempts to keep you engaged beyond the final tuck-in. Children can be masterful at extending the bedtime process to maintain contact with you and avoid sleep. Watch out! Sometimes we identify their master plan only after we've fallen prey to it. We don't mean to imply that children are manipulative or even plan their attempts to delay bedtime. Often, they are merely engaging in behaviors that have worked for them in the past. We all do this, often unconsciously. To avoid reinforcing or initiating unwanted patterns, keep your bedtime tuck-ins short and sweet. Since you won't be lingering and cuddling during the bedtime tuck-in, it is critical that you make time for that parent-child connection prior to bedtime (see parenting strategy number 2 above).

Here's a script for saying goodnight (we're keeping it both short and sweet *and* warm and firm): *It's time for bed now. I'm looking forward to seeing you in the morning. I love you! Goodnight.*

6. Use Planned Ignoring

It is natural for children to often seek out connection with their parents and find it incredibly rewarding to receive parental attention. Children sometimes seek connection with their parent in a manner that parents find inappropriate or disruptive. One way to reduce or eliminate this unwanted behavior is to use planned ignoring. Planned ignoring involves paying no attention to a child who is misbehaving (i.e., not doing what we want them to do). Some critics of this strategy purport that ignoring a child who is seeking attention can harm child mental health or the parent-child connection. Yet it is appropriate to use planned ignoring on certain occasions, such as when a child engages in minimally or moderately problematic behaviors such as repeatedly getting out of bed to go to the bathroom or making silly noises when they should be sleeping. Children don't experience psychological harm when parents require them to do things that are developmentally appropriate (e.g., requiring a child to refrain from intentionally making silly noises at night). So be sure that what you are requiring of your child is appropriate to their age, physical abilities, and developmental level. You can teach your child to *ask* for the desired attention to reduce the reliance on planned ignoring. Planned ignoring should never be used in response to unsafe behaviors (e.g., hitting, biting, destroying things), when your child is experiencing particularly strong emotions, or genuinely needs your help.

Successful use of this strategy might take some work on your part. We know how hard it can be to ignore some unwanted child behaviors, and children seem to always know which ones get your goat the most! Also, once you begin to ignore the unwanted behavior, be prepared for it to actually *increase* short-term. This is called an extinction burst. It occurs because the behavior got your attention in the past. Rest assured, continued planned ignoring will cause your child to give up that behavior because it no longer has the intended effect—getting your attention. For example, if your child repeatedly calls out from their bedroom at night, ignoring their calls (provided your child is in no real danger) will result in your child eventually giving up the behavior because it is no longer effective in beckoning you to their bedside.

Don't abandon the strategy too early assuming it is ineffective, especially once those unwanted behaviors temporarily increase. Stay the course and, with time, your child will stop engaging in the unwanted behaviors because they just don't work. Old habits die hard so give your child enough time to learn that the old way is no longer effective at producing the desired outcome. Planned ignoring is an effective parenting strategy that you will likely pull out of your parenting toolbox quite a bit to eliminate minor but unwanted child behaviors as your child grows.

7. Improve Your Own Ability to Tolerate Your Child's Discomfort

A happy child helps make for a happy parent, but to be a good parent, we need to look out for our children's best interests, even when doing so may cause them some discomfort. Imagine a child who is fearful of being sucked down the bathtub drain when the water is let out. Allowing your child to be distressed as the water runs down the drain (with you nearby uttering words of support and confidence) will ultimately allow your child to overcome this fear. A few drained bathtubs and your child will have learned that their worst fears were not realized. Better yet, they will have learned that they can face and conquer situations which make them nervous, and they will have sharpened their coping skills and emerged with a greater belief in their ability to handle tough situations. When you are faced with having to tolerate your child's discomfort, remember that you are giving your child the opportunity to develop strong coping skills, build their self-competence and confidence, and show them that you believe in their ability to handle challenging situations.

8. Selectively withhold Reassurance from Your Child

A natural parental inclination is to comfort your child when they are in distress. Yet doing so often makes the child's request for reassurance more likely to occur again and can diminish their self-competence. If your child continually and repeatedly asks for reassurance (e.g., Do you love me? Is this safe? Are the doors locked? Am I okay?), it may be very difficult to control your response. Though providing reassurance may *seem* supportive and loving, it reinforces (i.e., strengthens) the child's behavior, sends a message that their fear or concern is realistic, and confirms the child's belief they are unable to cope unless you respond. We won't ever ask you to stop all parental reassurances—just hold back on those that are excessive, overly repetitive, and reinforce anxious thinking. When your child asks you a reassurance-seeking question, empathize with them and their concerns: *You're feeling worried about something bad happening tonight . . . That must be hard to think about. What do you think is most likely to happen?* Or, *If that were to happen, what could you do about it?* This kind of response allows your child to feel heard and teaches them how to reassure themselves!

9. Implement Reward System

We often encounter parents who object to the notion of rewarding their child with toys, activities, experiences, or money for desired behaviors. These parents want their child to engage in desired behaviors without the expectation of such a reward. We do too! Yet rewarding (or positively reinforcing) a child's behavior is critical when shaping desired behaviors. This can often be achieved with praise, which is a valuable reward to which most parents don't object. When you want your child to agree to work hard on a major challenge, however, upgrading the reward incentive to activities, experiences, or even toys (monetary rewards are unnecessary) can make a big difference, though we don't support their use for the long-term.

Once the child's desired behavior has been occurring consistently, the reward is no longer necessary to keep the behavior in place. Most positive behaviors are rewarding enough in their own right to keep them going. Think of your own experiences with exercising. You may need some rewards to get started (stopping at the smoothie bar after a workout), but eventually the natural rewards associated with exercise (e.g., strength, energy, better sleep) become enough to sustain the behavior.

Setting up a reward system involving an activity, experience, or toy works like this: the child is given an incentive such as the possibility of earning some reward for engaging in a desired behavior, then the child engages in the desired behavior, and the child earns the reward. Thus, the child receives a reward for the effort they made to master the new (desired) behavior. For example, some children will require multiple prompts to begin the bedtime routine. In this case, parents should explain that if the child responds to the request with no more than one reminder, the child and parent will celebrate together in the morning (e.g., a high five, quick card game, or breakfast picnic on the living room floor). If the child doesn't respond until the third or fourth request, no reward will be bestowed, and the child will be encouraged to respond more immediately in the future. Once the child independently begins (and completes) the bedtime routine, parental praise and the child's sense of accomplishment should be sufficient to keep the behavior going.

10. Allow for Some Flexibility

Being flexible, or adaptable to change, is a life skill. You know what they say about the best-laid plans. Flexibility will undoubtedly be required for any child's bedtime routine. As with most things in life, we want to have a structured plan, but be prepared for the unexpected and be willing to adapt as needed. By allowing for some degree of flexibility during a structured bedtime routine, you're reducing stress for all involved and teaching your child how to adapt to change—essential in an unpredictable world!

When life requires you to temporarily adjust your child's routine (e.g., start the routine late, eliminate a portion of the routine, do things in an alternate order), be sure to communicate clearly to your child the circumstances that are necessitating this change and the temporary nature of the change (e.g., for one night, or only while on vacation). This clarity will remove any ambiguity about what will happen on subsequent nights, thus, greatly reducing the likelihood of future bedtime battles.

These ten key parenting strategies, specifically selected for their relevance to your child's independent sleep and delivered in a warm and firm manner, will also help to improve your child's overall functioning, not just their bedtime behavior. Now that you are armed with the tools and strategies for best assisting your child to sleep on their own, let's define the bedtime battle you are facing.

IDENTIFY YOUR CURRENT BEDTIME BATTLE

Below are some of the most common bedtime battles parents face. Because this book will offer a tailored approach to solving bedtime challenges, consider which bedtime battle(s) most closely approximates those you face. Strategies specific to each type of bedtime battle will be suggested in Week 5 so the intervention will be well suited to your child. Be sure to read through all of the bedtime battles because you may find that more than one applies to your child's nighttime difficulties. Identify your battle from the list below.

The Host

My child sleeps only if I lie with them in their bed or remain nearby until they fall asleep.

This can be a time-consuming and inconvenient routine depending on how long it takes your child to fall asleep. Like most parents, you've tried to send them to bed alone but that resulted in a temper tantrum for which you were no match. You've tried to sneak out of the bed before your child was fully asleep, but your child roused, begged you to stay, and you had to start the whole process over again. You've even unintentionally fallen asleep in your child's bed countless times. The problems abound! This particular bedtime battle may have origins in separation anxiety, a fear of the dark, or a combination of these. Some parents tell us that they lie with their child until sleep onset because they feel guilty about being so busy or otherwise occupied at other times of the day. Regardless of its origin, the plan we'll present to you is designed to help your child fall asleep on their own, increasing your child's independence and self-competence.

The Roommate
My child goes to sleep in my bed, and I must lie with them or remain nearby until they fall asleep.

There is no doubt that you are highly motivated to correct this cumbersome sleeping routine. Common pitfalls are numerous. You've tried to sneak out of the bed or the room because you don't share the same bedtime as your child, but your child wakes up and expresses concern over your departure. You've unintentionally fallen asleep while putting your child to bed. You manage to sneak away after your child is asleep, only to come to bed later in the evening to find your child sleeping spread eagle, requiring you to contort yourself while crawling into bed to avoid waking them. Your sleep is disrupted due to your child's multiple sleep positions and movements during the night. Your bed partner decides that there is not enough room for three people in a bed designed for two and has moved to the couch or guest bed. Like The Host, this bedtime battle may have origins in separation anxiety, fear of the dark, parental guilt about not being as present or available at other times of the day, or some combination of these. Regardless of the origin, easier nights lie ahead! You're here, taking the necessary steps toward positive change.

The Bed Warmer
My child goes to sleep on their own in my bed. They either stay there until I take them to their own bed or they stay in my bed all night.

This routine seemed harmless at first but now you dream of having your space all to yourself again. Parents who endure this sleep pattern have surely had to decide between carrying or leading their child to their own bed once they're asleep or gingerly getting into bed to avoid waking the child—a choice that most parents would rather not make. This bedtime battle may have origins in separation anxiety, fear of the dark, or both. Fortunately, regardless of the specific origin of this bedtime battle, you and your child will soon be snoozing in your respective bedrooms in peace.

The Demander
My child protests or has tantrums when told to begin their bedtime routine or to get into bed.

No matter how tired they are, how enticing their bed may be, or how little they are actually missing out on by going to bed, your child battles bedtime itself. Your child insists on doing bedtime their way—demanding extra time before bed, skipping over disliked elements of the bedtime routine (e.g., brushing their teeth), or insisting on having additional books read to them. This is a common bedtime battle, so know that you are not alone. This bedtime battle is often associated with oppositional behavior patterns or plain old strong will in your child. Once you "win" this bedtime battle, your child will be appreciative (though they may not actually show it!). There's no doubt that they, too, wish bedtime were easier.

The Curtain Caller
After being tucked in for the night, my child calls out, gets out of bed multiple times with complaints and requests, makes a lot of noise, or joins me in my bed (with or without my knowledge) one or more times during the night.

Getting your child to bed in the first place is tough enough, never mind the persistent requests for water or complaints about being unable to sleep. The energy that goes into responding to these complaints and requests is tremendous, leaving you frustrated and exhausted. This pattern of child behavior is strengthened each time you give in and fulfill the child's multiple requests, usually in search of a peaceful night's rest. Your child may be unable to remain quietly in bed for a host of reasons, usually not just one. In addition to reclaiming your evening, helping your child to learn to fall asleep on their own and in their own bed sends a message to your child that you're confident in their ability to fall asleep independently.

The Ritualizer

My child seems to obsess over going to bed at a certain time and becomes anxious if they're "behind schedule," or they have difficulty falling asleep if certain bedtime conditions are not present (e.g., a certain movie, song, or pillow arrangement).

This issue often baffles parents who cannot understand why their child is so intent on following their bedtime routine to a T. At first, you might have praised your child's obedience in following the bedtime rules, and you find their insistence on sticking to schedules and routines to be suggestive of their diligence and respect. After some time, however, you've begun to wonder whether this insistence on a strict routine might hold your child back. After all, daily life often brings unexpected events that require flexibility, compromise, and creativity. You may be concerned about your child's inability to manage the distress associated with changes, even small ones.

Like other bedtime battles, there's no single explanation for why some children experience this difficulty. These children may feel out of control in other areas of life or may have issues related to a developmental disability or obsessive-compulsive disorder (OCD). If you are concerned that your child might have an undiagnosed developmental disability or OCD, consult a licensed child psychologist or seek a neuropsychological evaluation for your child. Rest assured, this guide contains information that will undoubtedly be applicable to your parenting and to your child.

Helping a child with a reliance on rituals may seem as easy as following a strict bedtime routine, but alas, that may be considered accommodation and therefore a problem. In Week 5, we will guide you through steps to help your child be more flexible. Most often, this translates to increased flexibility in daytime activities as well, making things a whole lot easier for you and your child. It's a win-win!

IMPLEMENTING YOUR NEW BEDTIME ROUTINE
Set a Date to Start the Plan

You may decide to start the new plan in Week 5 or wait to use an upcoming milestone (e.g., your child's birthday, the start of the school year) as the starting date. Once decided, the start date should be nonnegotiable and, once begun, there should be no turning back. As we noted in Week 1, reverting to old routines makes things more difficult when you try again to have your child sleep independently. So as you select your date, check your child's calendar and your own. Be sure that your own schedule is not packed with important events demanding too much of your time and attention. Let the countdown begin!

Talk to Your Child about Upcoming Bedtime Changes

Now that you have identified the specific type of battle(s) you are facing and have chosen a start date, let's turn our attention to getting your child ready for the changes to come. When we introduce the notion of change to the bedtime routine, we want to do so in a manner that will lead to success. The best approaches are ones that are positively framed—highlighting the positive gains (e.g., increased energy, sense of accomplishment, self- and parental pride) that will come from independent sleep rather than discussing the things that will no longer occur or, from your child's perspective, are "lost" (e.g., co-sleeping, control over the timing or sequencing of the bedtime routine). It's best if you can get your child to approve of the process, though that is not required. Here, the work is yours. You should present the upcoming changes with a positive frame regardless of your child's reaction. Some children will cheerfully go along with change; others will not. No matter. Present the upcoming changes warmly and firmly.

Below is a sample script. Choose a time when your child is calm and able to give you their full attention.

> *Let's talk for a few minutes about sleep.* (Ask your child what they know about sleep.) *Sleep is super important in helping us to feel good and have the energy to do things we want and need to do. It gives our body a break after a long day of work and play. It helps our brains to remember what we learned and cleans out what we don't need so we can make room for new information! Sleep also helps us to feel pleasant, refreshed, and easy-going. You've seen me when I haven't gotten enough sleep, right? Yikes! So I know of some things we can do differently to help us to get better sleep.*
>
> *In addition to practicing mindful deep breathing and muscle relaxation, we're going to be making some more changes that will help you feel comfortable and independent at bedtime and will result in better sleep. Now that you're getting older, you have the privilege of getting to do more things on your own, like going to bed. Going to bed on your own will cut back on the squabbles we sometimes get in, improve your sleep, and leave you feeling really great. We're going to make these changes together and when we accomplish them, we'll celebrate! We're going to get started on* (insert start day here).

If you need a little encouragement prior to the "talk," here's some convincing data from recent research: Educating children about why sleep is so important and how to improve it resulted in a host of positive outcomes, including more sleep, better grades in math and English, better emotional control, and less impulsivity. Even more amazing, these improvements were seen with only small increases (as few as twenty to thirty minutes) in the duration of sleep![3] If your child appears interested in sleep, feel free to share more of the details that you read about in Week 1. It's never too early to arm your child with information that will impress upon them the importance of sleep and inspire them to give more and higher quality sleep a try.

In reviewing the upcoming changes, be certain to allow your child time for questions and concerns and to make reasonable suggestions to the plan. Clear communication is essential! Excitement and motivation can be built by reading children's books on the topics of developing independence and self-competence and sleeping on one's own. See table 4.1 for a few of our favorites that you can find at your local library.

Older children may also be motivated by recognition of the benefits that will occur once they can sleep on their own—think not only of sleepovers and travel with friends and family, but also of increased self-confidence and a feeling of mastery over something difficult.

Whether your child is younger or older, it is important to validate their desire to sleep with you; show them that you understand how important that feeling of closeness is and assure them that it will not be lost. Take the time to thoroughly and clearly explain why your expectations for them are changing, taking care to listen intently to their thoughts and concerns, while sending the message that the decision is final and not up for debate.

Ask your child, "What's making it hard for you to sleep in your room?" and then see if you can problem-solve some of the issues without giving up on the main goal of getting them to sleep independently. If your child can't identify or express what makes it scary or difficult, offer up some of the common concerns of children: being alone, intruders, unidentified sounds, monsters, feeling vulnerable to "the dark," fear of what will happen if they can't sleep, fear of missing out on parents' or siblings' activities. Presenting options from which to choose ("is it any of these common concerns?") can help children to understand their fears and help you to correct any misperceptions your child may have.

Helping your child to identify what specifically makes them nervous or uncomfortable puts you in a better position to help

Table 4.1. Recommended Books to Read at Bedtime

Book	Recommended Age
I Will Be Fierce by Bea Birdsong	3–6 years
Ruby Finds a Worry by Tom Percival	3–6 years
I Can Do Hard Things: Mindful Affirmations for Kids by Gabi Garcia and Charity Russell	3–7 years
Dear Girl: A Celebration of Wonderful, Smart, Beautiful You by Amy Krouse Rosenthal and Paris Rosenthal	3–7 years
Patrick Picklebottom and the Penny Book by Mr. Jay	3–7 years
The Invisible String by Patrice Karst	3–8 years
My Bed: Enchanting Ways to Fall Asleep around the World by Rebecca Bond and Salley Mavor	4–7 years
Outside In by Deborah Underwood	4–7 years
Bedtime Meditation for Kids: Quick Calming Exercises to Help Kids Get to Sleep by Cory Cochiolo	4–8 years
Tengo un Nudo en la Barriga by B de Blok	4–8 years
What Do You Do with a Problem? by Kobi Yamada	4–8 years
What's in Your Mind Today? by Louise Bladen	4–8 years
What the Road Said by Cleo Wade	5–13 years
Worry Says What by Allison Edwards	5–13 years
Uncle Lightfoot, Flip That Switch: Overcoming Fear of the Dark by Mary Coffman	8–12 years
Outsmarting Worry: An Older Kid's Guide to Managing Anxiety by Dawn Huebner	9–13 years

them think through the unlikelihood of that worry coming true. A little bit of clarity and information can often go a long way toward easing nighttime fears. For example, understanding that as homes and buildings age or "cool down" during the night, their structural materials (e.g., wood, window glass, nails) and mechanical systems (e.g., plumbing, heating) can move slightly, sometimes rubbing against one another and making the creaks and pops that we may hear.

If your child is unable to verbalize their specific concern or fear, that's okay. Knowing everything that makes your child uncomfortable or scared at night is not essential—your child's fears will fade as you begin the new sleep plan, and they learn that they can rely on their own coping skills to manage their emotions.

If necessary, remind your child that, as a parent, it is your responsibility to make choices and decisions that are in their best interest, even when these decisions are difficult or cause them fear or distress in the short-term. To reiterate the words of a wise psychologist mom, "We do hard things in order to learn how to do hard things." Highlight the pride that your child will feel. It's not important that your child is happy with your decision. It is important, however, that they feel heard and understood and that you communicate your decision and the rationale behind it. Acknowledge your child's feelings, validate that change is hard, and stay the course (warm and firm). You can say something to the effect of: *I understand this will be difficult for you at first, but it will get easier over time. That's usually how it goes when we do hard things. I know you can do this! I believe in you!*

Once these components have been discussed, refrain from rehashes and debates. Ignore your child's attempts to cajole or otherwise convince you to change your mind. These discussions are almost always unproductive, especially when they occur at night or in the midst of big emotions.

Create a Title of Honor for Your Child

To boost motivation (and pride), it's fun to come up with a catchy "title" your child can earn for mastering independent sleep. For example, perhaps your child will become "Sleep Master of the Universe," "Sleeper of the Year," a "Sleep Superhero," or a "Sleeping Princess." Get your child involved in finding the title that is most fun and inspiring! Perhaps a family contest for the catchiest title is in order. Have fun with this. Perhaps the "Sleeping Princess" wears a special crown at breakfast the morning after a night of independent sleep!

Develop a Reward System

Next, discuss appropriate rewards for the difficult work that you and your child are going to do. Rewards should be provided in a timely fashion, inexpensive, and scaled in size to match the effort expended by your child. Rewards can include stickers or points that are redeemed for toys or fun activities. You can use posters, charts, or other creative means to display the rewards and points earned. Be sure that you are clear about precisely what behavior merits the reward. It is most effective to reward one or two behaviors at a time. Over the span of a few weeks, you can make the reward contingent on a sequence of behaviors. Do not deduct points or remove stickers for unwanted behaviors.

This system works best when the reward is inexpensive (or free), is delivered immediately following the desired behavior, and can be adjusted to the size of the goal (e.g., five stickers = choosing dessert for the family, ten stickers = a trip to the park). Parents are often surprised that their children can be motivated by low-cost or no-cost rewards; yet we've found they can be extremely effective in motivating change.

The delivery of the reward should occur with meaningful praise ("Congratulations on sleeping in your bed all night! Let's add two stickers to the chart we made"). When the reward is not achieved, news of the absence of the reward should be delivered matter-of-factly and without shame, criticism, embarrassment, or punishment to the child ("You didn't earn a reward today, but you can try again tomorrow"). Let your child know that they shouldn't be afraid of challenges and that their attempt is just the first attempt in learning. Sometimes learning to do something new can take multiple attempts. We like to remind children who get focused on failure that "FAIL" is nothing more than a First Attempt In Learning!

You can access a blank Reward Chart at the end of this week's reading. We've listed some examples of possible rewards in table 4.2 to get you started.

Also note that if you have a hard time sticking to the plan, set up a reward program for yourself! Remember that this is difficult work that requires a lot of your effort too.

Add a Special Touch to the Bedroom

For a final flourish of excitement, consider making a special change to your child's bedroom, such as repositioning the furniture, purchasing a special pillow or colorful sheets, or painting a wall in the room. Adding that special touch at the onset of the plan can add to your child's overall enthusiasm for the plan. But don't add the special touches until it's go time (Week 5). As you may have noticed yourself, the shine of new items can rub off quickly, and we want that momentum on our side.

Ready, Set . . .

Next week, you will be learning the final steps to take to turn your child into an independent sleeper. Because your child will, more than likely, be opposed to the new nighttime changes, it is important that you move to the next phase when you are able to devote significant time and attention to the change. You may get less sleep. Your child may be more disagreeable. In fact, be prepared

Table 4.2. List of Appropriate and Effective Rewards to Support Child Behavior Change

Reward Ideas
Playtime at favorite (or new) playground
Playdate
Trip to museum or movies
Special parent-child activity (e.g., painting, biking, catch)
Bedroom updates such as new wall paint color or decor
Choice of dinner or dessert for the family
Choice of game or movie on a family night
Token reward (stickers or points) to redeem for a new game
Exemption from chores for a day, days, or a week
Rights to preferred seating or other arrangements for a day/week (e.g., on couch, in car, at dining table)
Scavenger hunt
Camping in backyard
Breakfast in bed
Reverse bedtime—the kid puts the parent to bed at bedtime (and then puts themselves to bed)
Grab bag surprise
Sleeping with family pet
Helping to bake cookies
New book or magazine

for the real possibility of a worsening of your child's nighttime misbehavior. Once you firmly set the new bedtime routine, your child may push back, doubling and tripling their efforts to resist the new changes. If such outbursts have led you to give in in the past, your child is especially likely to protest strongly, loudly, and more fiercely than ever before. This is entirely normal behavior for a child. Hold the line with your child, and the protesting behavior will disappear once your child sees how serious you are about upholding the new plan. Giving in or giving up at this point will make future attempts to get your child sleeping independently even more difficult. So proceed to Week 5 only when you are ready.

Now Apply It!

1. Talk with your child about the upcoming plan for independent sleep. Once you've prepared the sleep environment, select a firm start date, find a fitting title for your child, and make some fun changes to the room to create excitement and motivation!

2. Working with your child, develop a reward system that is sustainable for your family. Use the Reward Chart* provided or make your own.

3. Continue practice in mindful breathing, progressive muscle relaxation, and cognitive restructuring.

*Access the Reward Chart by scanning the QR code below or by going to www.highperformance-parenting .com/bbb-appendices.

WEEK 4 SUMMARY

- In a warm and firm parenting style, use the following ten key parenting strategies for improving bedtime:
- Clearly communicate your expectations for the new bedtime routine, not only as you introduce the plan but also as you implement it.
- Ritualize parent-child snuggle time and keep snuggling in your child's bed to a reasonable timeframe. If necessary,

move the snuggling to another time and location to reduce interference with your child's independent sleep.

- Support your child's use of emotional control strategies by teaching them calming techniques they can use on their own.

- Use shaping to help your child get closer and closer to the end goal.

- Limit the length and number of interactions between you and your child post-bedtime to promote independent sleep.

- Use planned ignoring as appropriate to eliminate unwanted child behaviors.

- Learn to tolerate your child's discomfort. Allowing your child to be mildly distressed provides them opportunities to learn to manage it.

- Avoid excessive reassurance to steer clear of reinforcing unreasonable fears and worries.

- Use a reward system to motivate your child and support their independent sleep efforts.

- Allow for occasional flexibility in the bedtime routine. Doing so will build your child's ability to tolerate and overcome the discomfort that often comes with change.

- Identify the specific bedtime battle(s) that you most commonly face.

- Set a date to begin the new bedtime plan.

- Talk to your child about the new bedtime plan using the sample script as a guide. Be sure to highlight the benefits associated with the upcoming changes.

- Read a book with your child about independence, learning to do new things, and sleeping on one's own. See table 4.1 for a few recommended books.

- Create a title of honor for your child, develop the reward system, and add a special touch to the bedroom.

You're Ready, Set, Go!

OKAY, IT'S FINALLY HERE—GO TIME! THE WEEK YOU'VE BEEN waiting for. The week when you will implement your child's new bedtime plan. You've set the stage and now your plan is put to the test. You and your child will be put to the test as well. Keep your eye on the long-term benefits. Children who use bedtime routines to get sufficient sleep see lifelong advantages, including better self-care and health practices, improved literacy and language development, improved parent and family functioning, and enhanced emotional and behavioral regulation. You can make a difference across a wide range of child behaviors with this one parenting move. Get set for the parenting win!

Read the entirety of Week 5 prior to implementing your child's new bedtime plan.

You will be making gradual changes to your child's current bedtime routine as you transition to the new routine. These gradual changes will likely occur in a step-like fashion. For example, for a child who watches videos every night to "relax," you might design a step-by-step transition plan in which your child shifts from watching just any videos to video-guided relaxation exercises, to parent-guided relaxation exercises, to self-guided relaxation exercises. These small steps are key to keeping your child's anxiety or distress low enough to make measured and continued progress toward the goal of independent sleep.

Keep track of the steps you and your child decide upon as you move from the old routine to the new bedtime plan using the Step-by-Step Transition Plan worksheet. This will keep you organized in working toward the goal. You can access it at the end of this week's reading.

The timing associated with the implementation of the new plan is up to you. There are two approaches. Option 1: Move from your child's current routine to the new routine via a process called fading—you *gradually* drop the old routine in favor of the new routine. Option 2: Set a date for the initiation of the new routine and switch to the new routine *all at once*. The old routine is out and the new routine is in! While there is no correct option here, we have a strong preference for option 1. A gradual transition to the new routine tends to be far easier on parents and children alike. However, if your child tends to prefer to jump into things to get them over with (think of jumping into a pool on a hot day versus getting into the shallow end to slowly become acclimated to the water) or if you need to make the bedtime changes quickly, you might opt for option 2.

Ensure that your plan fits your family's needs, is reasonable, and be certain that you (and any parenting partners or other relevant family members) are ready for and committed to this change. Let's briefly review elements of a good bedtime plan that you should consider as you implement your plan.

A few reminders:

1. Keep the bedtime routine to about thirty minutes. Ensure that everyone, especially your child, knows the time to start the routine as well as the time that they should be in bed.

2. Limit technology use in the hours leading up to the bedtime routine and consider removing all electronic devices from

the bedroom during the nighttime hours. If the electronic devices are not removed, ensure that they are kept far from the bed at night.

3. Limit light as much as possible and keep the bedroom cool.

4. Be aware of sleep associations (things that your child pairs with falling asleep, like your presence, a certain smell, or a favorite stuffed animal). These items, people, or conditions can serve to help your child fall asleep in the short-run but can hinder their ability to sleep independently in the long-run. The only association that we really want to support is the association between your child's bed and your child's sleep! So if you are planning the continued use of sleep aids (e.g., melatonin supplements, fan, night-light), be sure to phase them out over time and certainly don't introduce any new ones. You can wait until the routine is firmly established and your child is sleeping well. Then, using a gradual approach, decrease the amount, the time, or the use of the sleep aid until it is no longer needed.

5. Don't forget about the effects of caffeine and other foods that can disrupt sleep. Select bedtime snacks that are sleep-promoting.

6. Be warm and firm with your child as you start the new bedtime plan. Take on a cheerful and supportive demeanor that is encouraging. Let your child know that you believe in their ability to sleep independently and that you are excited to see them develop their independence. The goal of this week is to begin to teach your child to fall asleep on their own.

YOUR TAILORED PLAN
Below you will find each type of battle paired with instructions for achieving independent sleep and a sample vignette for illustration. Find the battle(s) you face to discover the plan that's tailored to

your child's bedtime behaviors. Alternatively, read them all to be prepared for any bedtime behavior problems that may come your way!

The Host

My child sleeps only if I lie with them in their bed or remain nearby until they fall asleep.

With this battle, you'll be gradually removing yourself from needing to be with your child as they fall to sleep. While this sounds like one goal, you are really working on two goals here. Goal 1: to gradually decrease the amount of time you spend in the presence of your child while your child is in bed but still awake (decreasing time). Goal 2: to gradually move yourself farther and farther from your child after they lie down for sleep (increasing distance). Your child has most likely become dependent upon your presence to fall asleep. In short, your presence has become *required* for their sleep.

To establish healthy sleeping habits, it will be important for your child to fall asleep on their own. Since it may have been a very long time since your child has done this, it will be best to ease into this gradually. To facilitate your child's ability to fall asleep independently, decrease your time in the child's presence at bedtime and increase your distance from your child as they are transitioning from being awake to asleep.

Over the course of a week or two, decrease your time by removing yourself from your child's presence when

1. Your child is *very close to sleep.*

2. Your child is only *beginning to get drowsy.*

3. Your child is *tucked in and settled but not yet drowsy.*

Simultaneously, increase your distance by gradually moving farther away as your child is ready for sleep. The whole process should not take more than a few weeks.

1. Move yourself out of your child's bed to a nearby chair.

2. Shift that chair (or your position) farther and farther from your child's bed.

3. Position yourself in the doorway of your child's bedroom.

4. Move out of your child's bedroom and into a hallway, if needed, until you are completely out of your child's sight, and they are falling asleep without you.

While working toward these two goals, it is important to refrain from engaging with your child. We are encouraging them to settle down for the night and to learn to sleep on their own. Conversation and reassurances from you during this time will make it more difficult for your child to unwind and learn to sleep on their own.

Make no mistake, however—you should *not* give up the snuggles and bedtime closeness that many children and parents enjoy. We are working toward a bedtime tuck-in that is healthy for both you and your child. We want to establish a routine that enables your child to feel loved and secure and permits you to then leave the room to carry on with your own nighttime plans and routines.

Some families may wish to do a brief tuck-in in the child's bedroom (e.g., parent walks to child's bed with child, lies down or sits with them for five to ten minutes of in-the-bedroom parent-child interaction, and then leaves after a hug/kiss/saying "goodnight"). Other families may prefer to eliminate the bedtime tuck-in in favor of a pre-bedtime goodnight ritual (e.g., parent and child complete some out-of-the-bedroom parent-child interaction prior to the child independently heading to their bed to go to sleep). Keep in mind that there is no one right way to send your child off to sleep. If you follow the healthy sleeping recommendations we've laid out in this book, you and your child will be enjoying some serious shut-eye!

Vignette: The Host

For as long as she can remember, Mel has lain down with seven-year-old Harper in Harper's bed until she is fast asleep. Often, Mel also falls asleep! When Mel wakes several hours later, her grogginess makes any hope of catching up on work out of the question, and it is usually too late to engage in any pleasurable activities such as reading.

Mel fantasizes about a routine in which she tucks Harper into bed around 8:30 p.m. and then has some free time to herself. She's tried telling Harper to go to sleep on her own, but Harper protests and her pleas are hard to resist. Plus, Mel knows Harper will get to sleep faster if she just lies down with her. Mel tries mightily to resist falling asleep herself—sometimes she is successful, but most nights she wakes in Harper's bed in the wee hours of the morning.

After recognizing Harper's behavior in the description of The Host, Mel carefully follows the plan associated with that battle type. Mel introduces Harper to a new bedtime routine: "Starting this week, we are going to work together to change your bedtime routine. You're used to having me with you when you go to sleep, but it'll be better for everyone when you get used to going to sleep independently. It may seem difficult now but we're both in this together, and we'll make only small changes at a time. First, we're going to have our snuggle time on the couch at 7:45 p.m. We can read, play a quiet game, or just talk. Then, you're going to start getting ready for bed at 8 p.m. This means that at 8 p.m., you'll stop what you're doing, get changed into your PJs, brush your teeth, and wash your face. Of course, I'll still be here to make sure you don't forget. At 8:30 p.m., you'll get into your bed. I'll give you more and more time to yourself each night until you're comfortable falling asleep on your own. New routines are tough at first, but I know you can do it!"

In the days leading up to the independent sleep start date, Mel takes care to practice relaxation exercises chosen by Harper, and together, they do mindful deep breathing each night before bed. After a week or so, Mel has Harper take the lead in the relaxation exercises, prompting Harper to begin only when she has forgotten.

Mel and Harper kick off the first night of the new plan with reading, snuggling, and relaxation. Mel lies in bed with Harper, not until Harper falls asleep, but instead, she waits until Harper's breathing has slowed and sleep is very near. Then, Mel carefully gets out of Harper's bed and leaves the room. Harper remains nearly asleep and settled. Mel repeats this for three nights in a row. On the fourth night, instead of lying down with Harper, Mel creates more distance from Harper by sitting in a chair next to Harper's bed. She still leaves the room only once Harper is drowsy and nearly asleep.

After another few days, Mel moves the chair farther from Harper's bed. Although Harper protests, Mel gently reminds her daughter of her confidence in her ability to fall asleep on her own, holds firmly to the plan, and reminds Harper of the reward she is working toward earning. With the chair positioned even farther away from the bed, Mel now leaves the room when Harper is fully awake but settled in bed. Finally, Mel decides it's time to tuck Harper into bed, and then leave the room altogether after a brief hug and kiss. Harper calls out after her a few times but, using all her parental resolve, Mel doesn't answer (planned ignoring). In the morning, Mel and Harper talk about the callouts. Mel explains that while calling out or getting out of bed after bedtime used to be allowed and she understands why Harper did it, it is no longer allowed. The only exceptions are emergencies (e.g., fire, vomiting, bleeding, etc.). Mel follows through on the reward system that she and Harper agreed upon earlier in the week. Mel makes French toast for breakfast—Harper's favorite—and they eat it together on mornings that follow a successful night of independent sleep.

The Roommate

My child goes to sleep in my bed, and I must lie with them or remain nearby until they fall asleep.

Your first step will be to move your child's sleeping location from your bed (or bedroom floor) to a more suitable location. Typically, this is the child's own bed. Once that change has been made, the next step is to gradually decrease the reliance on your physical presence so that your child can fall asleep without you nearby. This is usually accomplished by increasing the physical distance between you and your child and decreasing the time you spend in their presence as they fall to sleep.

Let's start at the top—moving your child's sleeping location from your bedroom to their own. You may wish to do this in one night or more gradually across a week or two. Keep in mind that your child will still insist on your physical presence as they fall to sleep. Making the change in one night may result in more initial protests from your child but also has the advantage of (1) letting them know that you are serious about your expectations for change, (2) reducing their ability to finagle or negotiate during the change of sleeping location, (3) reducing your child's discomfort or anxiety since you will still be staying close to your child as they fall asleep, and (4) getting your child to sleep independently more quickly.

If you choose to have your child move more gradually, have them move from your bed to a sleeping bag or blanket on the floor next to your bed. Then, have them move farther away from your bed. Ultimately, you can move the sleeping bag or blanket into locations that move progressively from your bedroom and into your child's bedroom. You don't want to continue this process for more than a week or two. It has the potential to make the change more difficult for all involved—even though the change in sleeping location would be more gradual, the overall process of change would be drawn out longer.

Once your child is sleeping in their bedroom, your next goal is to allow your child to fall asleep without you nearby. Since it may have been a long time since your child has fallen asleep on their own, it will be best to ease into this gradually. First, you may stay near to your child (as you have been) while staying silent and refraining from engaging with your child, but leave the room when your child becomes noticeably drowsy and is just about asleep. If your child cannot tolerate this, rousing and becoming upset when you move to leave the room, try instead to put some distance between you and your child, rather than leaving the room entirely. So if you are currently lying in your child's bed with them until they are fast asleep, you might increase your distance by moving to a chair placed next to the bed when you see that your child is close to sleep. Remember the importance of remaining quiet and refraining from conversation and other engagement with your child as you sit in the chair and your child lies down to sleep. Then, in a gradual step-like fashion, continue to leave earlier and earlier over the next days and weeks.

So the rollout is the following: first, you create physical distance (by leaving the bedroom altogether or moving some distance away from the bed) when your child is *very close to sleep*. Next, you create physical distance (or leave the bedroom) when your child is *beginning to get drowsy*. Then, you might create physical distance after your child is *tucked in and settled*. You can see that we are working to both (1) gradually allow your child more and more time to grow accustomed to falling asleep by themselves, and (2) eliminate the need for you to be physically close for extended periods of time during the bedtime routine.

It is not uncommon for children to wake in the middle of the night and return to their preferred sleeping environment (in this case, with you in your bed). Your efforts in teaching your child to fall to sleep without you present is key in moving past these middle-of-the-night visits. If your child hasn't learned to fall asleep on their own, then every middle-of-the-night awakening will require your presence for your child to return to sleep. If, instead, your child becomes used to falling asleep alone, a middle-of-the-night awakening becomes no big deal. Your child can return to sleep without you.

If you have a middle-of-the-night visitor, do the following: calmly and quietly escort them back to their bed and leave their bedroom immediately. You'll risk setting the whole process back if you lie down or stay with your child until they fall back to sleep. If your child calls out to you from their bed, use planned ignoring to stop the unwanted behavior. Be sure that your child understands that calling out in the middle of the night is not permitted and that you will not respond to them if they call out. Soon your child will learn that the middle-of-the night trips (or callouts) to your bedroom are not effective in convincing you to allow them back into your bed for the night or getting you to stay with them as they fall asleep in their bed. Once that message is received, your child will give up the midnight escapades. It is also helpful to point out to your child that you have great confidence in their ability to sleep on their own. If necessary, you can give your child some guidelines about when it is appropriate to get out of bed or to call out in the middle of the night (e.g., vomiting, bleeding, fire, or other emergency). Be sure that you clearly define what is meant by an "emergency" (e.g., being thirsty is not an emergency).

Vignette: The Roommate

Catherine and her ex share custody of their six-year-old son, Manny. She has Manny every other week. Catherine misses him terribly when he's not staying with her. Thus, when Manny stays at her house, she does everything she can to maximize her time with him, including lying down with him in her bed at night. Manny won't let her leave until he has fallen asleep, and she'd feel guilty if she did. So it's become a persistent pattern. Not wanting to miss a moment with Manny, Catherine waits to do the dishes, watch the evening news, and catch up on work-related tasks until after Manny is asleep. This makes for a very late night, and Catherine is feeling the effects of chronic sleep loss. She feels groggy during the day and is worried that her work performance may be affected. Even her friend commented that she seemed "off" over the last few weeks. Catherine's concerns prompt her to rethink Manny's bedtime routine. She decides to reclaim her bed and help Manny feel more confident and comfortable with sleeping in his own bedroom.

Catherine recognizes that Manny's behaviors are consistent with those described in The Roommate and prepares to follow the recommendations for that particular battle type. She starts by referencing the ideal bedtime routine she created for Manny several weeks prior, in Weeks 1 and 3. Catherine doesn't want to lose the closeness that she and Manny share when they lie together at night, so she decides to shift the time and place of those snuggles. Catherine decides to have snuggle time on the couch at 7:15 p.m. before Manny's 8 p.m. bedtime. Desiring to make the transition as quick as possible, Catherine plans first to shift Manny's sleeping location to his own bed and out of hers. She then will gradually reduce her time with Manny in his room as he gets ready to fall asleep.

Catherine takes the time to explain the upcoming bedtime changes: "Starting this week, we're going to work together to make your bedtime routine go more smoothly. You're used to sleeping with me in my bed, but it'll be better for both of us when you get used to sleeping in your own bed and on your own. First, we'll make the switch from my bed to yours. Then, I'm going to give you more and more time to yourself until you're comfortable falling asleep on your own. We're in this together, and we will only make small changes at a time." Manny is doubtful about his ability to adjust to the changes. Catherine acknowledges his concerns and remains firm about the plan.

On night one, Catherine and Manny start off in Manny's bed. Catherine leads Manny through the progressive muscle relaxation exercise. She plans to have Manny take the lead on the relaxation routine over the next days, reminding him to do it only when he's forgotten. She leaves Manny's bedroom ten minutes after the relaxation exercises are completed and Manny is close to drifting off to sleep.

Over the course of the next two weeks, she leaves Manny's bedroom earlier and earlier to allow him the practice of falling asleep on his own—first leaving ten minutes after the relaxation exercises, then five minutes after, and then immediately after.

Catherine follows through on the reward system she established to recognize Manny's efforts and promote continued participation in this new routine. Manny earns the seat at the head of the dining table on mornings that follow a successful night of independent sleep, an honor that Manny finds exciting.

The Bed Warmer

My child goes to sleep on their own in my bed. They either stay there until I take them to their own bed or they stay in my bed all night.

The good news is that your child can fall asleep on their own! This is a critical skill for independent sleeping, and therefore, your child has a leg up on the sleeping game. Three cheers for your child (and for you)! Your goal is to transition your child to a new sleeping environment—their own bed. Because your child can fall asleep without your presence, you should expect your child to have a bit of an easier time than children who need a parent nearby to fall asleep.

Initially, your child's transition from your bed to their bed will be made easier by encouraging your child to associate pleasant feelings with their bedroom. You'll want them to begin to feel comfortable in the space, spending time there during the day and, eventually, in the evening in preparation for the move back to their bed. Take care to encourage child activities that do not interfere with your child's associations between bed and sleep.

Once your child is at ease in their bedroom during the day and evening hours, you are ready to change their sleeping location. You can have your child move from your bed to their bed in one step (i.e., in one night) or alternatively, you can make a more gradual transition by having them first sleep in a sleeping bag (or blanket) on the floor of your bedroom, then having them move the sleeping bag closer and closer to their own bed before finally having them place it on their own bed! Voilà—done!

Because your child is accustomed to sleeping *in your bed*, and, for those children who stay in their parent's bed all night, sleeping *with you*, they may want to return to your bed if they wake in the middle of the night. Be prepared for this by clearly communicating the expectation that they are to stay in their bed all night long. If you have a middle-of-the-night visitor, calmly and quietly escort them back to their bed and leave their room immediately. Do this as many times as is necessary. You'll risk setting the whole process back if you lie down or stay with your child until they fall back to sleep.

If your child calls out to you from their bed, use planned ignoring to put an end to this unwanted behavior. Clearly communicate to your child (outside of sleeping hours) that yelling out in the middle of the night is not acceptable behavior and that you will not respond if they do. Soon your child will learn that calling out or visiting your bedroom in the middle of the night will not end up getting them what they want—sleeping in your bed or you sleeping in theirs. Once your child understands that their behaviors are not bringing them closer to what they want, they will give up the midnight visits and callouts. It is always a good idea to give your child guidelines about when it is appropriate to seek you out in the middle of the night (e.g., vomiting, bleeding, fire, or other emergency). You'll want to clearly define what is meant by an "emergency" (e.g., a fly buzzing around the bedroom is not an emergency).

Vignette: The Bed Warmer

Kyle and his nine-year-old daughter, Luisa, have fallen into a sleeping pattern in which Luisa falls asleep each night in Kyle's bed. Once Kyle is ready for bed, he gently carries his sleeping daughter to her own bed.

Luisa barely rouses during the late-night bed switcheroo. Kyle wants to be sure that Luisa feels safe and comfortable sleeping in her own bed, and he knows that he won't be able to carry her to her bed forever!

Kyle quickly recognizes his daughter's behaviors as fitting into *The Bed Warmer*, and he begins to follow the plan associated with that battle type. Kyle introduces the new bedtime plan to his daughter who receives the news with anxiety. To increase Luisa's comfort with being in her own room, Kyle has Luisa spend more time in her room during the day. During the week of the transition, Kyle facilitates play (board games) with Luisa in her bedroom after school. In addition, Kyle adds a brief period of reading to their bedtime routine to help Luisa develop some more positive bedroom associations, thus helping her to feel more comfortable in her bedroom at night.

Kyle and Luisa also decide on a reward system in which she can earn the privilege of selecting the game to play on family game night or going out for ice cream if she has slept independently for at least six out of seven nights. Because Kyle knows the importance of providing a reward near in time to Luisa's sleep success, he will also celebrate her achievement with their special secret handshake in the morning. Before the big day in which Luisa will sleep in her own bed, she and Kyle have some fun creating inspirational posters and confidence-boosting signs for her bedroom walls.

On the big day and each night following, Kyle tucks in Luisa at 8:30 p.m., her bedtime, and reads to her for fifteen minutes. Then, following a hug and kiss, he leaves the bedroom and goes downstairs to spend the remainder of the evening free to do as he wishes.

Since Luisa was already skilled at falling asleep on her own, the transition to falling asleep in her own room is a relatively smooth one.

The Demander
My child protests or has tantrums when told to begin their bedtime routine or to get into bed.

This plan is for those strong-willed children who protest and complain most nights when faced with the prospect of bedtime.

They may refuse silently or loudly, yet each night is a struggle. Bedtime has become a dreaded event for both you and your child, as it signals the start of a drawn-out battle of wills, and the side with the greatest endurance declares the evening's victory. Let's face it, your child has youth on their side so the win may often go in their column! The good news is that your child is persistent; the bad news is that your child is persistent.

Your goal is to teach your child to manage their distress (i.e., distress tolerance skills) and control their emotions (i.e., emotion regulation skills) using coping skills such as those presented in Week 3. In addition, you will want to set and enforce compliance with your expectations of them when it's bedtime. To do this, you'll need to clearly communicate your expectations for bedtime behaviors and implement a positive behavioral approach in which your child is rewarded for following the rules and expectations. If your child's behavior is wildly inappropriate or unsafe (e.g., hitting, jumping on the bed, throwing things), consequences may be imposed to deter similar behaviors in the future. Mildly unacceptable behaviors (e.g., eye rolling, muttering under breath) to moderately unacceptable behaviors (e.g., yelling, stomping) can be handled with planned ignoring (this technique was presented in Week 4).

As you respond to your child's misbehavior, use a neutral emotional expression (this will be hard!). Keeping your cool will help to prevent the situation from escalating. If one of two parties refuses to engage in the "fight," the other side has a very difficult time escalating it further. A colleague once told us about a Mark Twain quote he'd read on a placemat in a Texan restaurant: "Don't wrestle with a pig. You'll both get dirty, and the pig likes it." While we are not drawing a comparison between children and pigs, we find this quote a valuable instruction in managing conflict. When one refuses to wrestle, the fight can't continue and may never get started!

On the issue of clear expectations, you may be thinking, "But I already communicate my expectations for bedtime. I couldn't be clearer!" That may be true; however, have you tried communicating the expectations at a time other than bedtime, such as during the morning or another time when both your and your child's emotions are cool and steady?

Communicate to your child your concerns about the bedtime difficulties and express your wish to make it easier for them. Explain that they can earn rewards for following bedtime expectations and can help to select their reward. *Frame this as an exciting adventure, not as another rule to follow.* Remember, the reward *must be motivating* for it to be an effective tool for behavior change!

Depending on the reward, you may opt to use a tracking chart to keep track of both the desired behavior as well as the rewards (e.g., six successful bedtimes per week earns the child a visit to a local park). Alternatively, for every successful bedtime, your child may earn fifteen extra minutes of video game time the next day, which may be simpler to keep track of and may not necessitate a tracking chart.

Once your child is motivated to follow expectations, we must consider whether they have the skills to tolerate the distress that arises when they are directed to go to bed. They may become distressed due to any of the following reasons: they have way more fun playing video or other games than going to bed; they like getting the parental attention their distress evokes; they feel as if they're missing out on something fun once they go to bed; any combination of these, or something else entirely. Whichever it may be, use of "warm and firm" parenting applies. This translates to acknowledging and validating your child's feelings by saying to them, "You're really upset that it's already bedtime . . . sometimes I don't want to go to bed either." Next, bring on the *firm*: "And to earn your [insert reward here], you'll brush your teeth now."

If your child protests, even a little bit, they do not earn their reward or token for that evening. There should be no arguing about it. Just tell your child that tomorrow is another opportunity to try again. Use planned ignoring if the protesting continues. When your child eventually goes to bed (reluctantly or otherwise), praise them for doing so, and remind them that they have an opportunity to try again the next day.

Allowing for anger and disappointment when your child fails to earn the reward permits your child to learn to cope with distressing emotions. It is worth noting that there is an important distinction between emotions and behaviors. While it is perfectly acceptable for your child to *feel* angry, disappointed, and any other emotion, it is not acceptable for them to *behave* in ways that illustrate their intense negative emotions which may harm others (e.g., hitting, throwing objects). Far too often, parents are reluctant to provide consequences for their child's misbehavior because the misbehavior is born of a legitimate emotion ("I don't want to punish my child for their tantrums at bedtime because they are scared of sleeping alone"). All emotions are okay; all behaviors are not.

Avoid telling your child to stop being upset. It's unproductive and may lead to confusion and withdrawal. Imagine your boss tells you, "Stop feeling so frustrated—just get over it." Their response doesn't change the fact that you're frustrated, and it probably makes you feel worse. Imagine instead your boss says, "I sense your frustration. Can you tell me what you're thinking?" How would you feel? Seen? Understood? Bottom line, let your child experience their emotions, set limits on negative behaviors, and encourage healthy emotional expression.

Take the case of a child who feels angry about having to go to bed earlier than their older sibling. The child is entitled to their anger and should be allowed to express it but may not do so by engaging in misbehavior (e.g., hitting, yelling). Parents must help to support the expression of all emotions, even unpleasant ones, so long as the emotional expression is healthy. For example, the parent may say, "You look like you're upset, but you cannot throw things. Let's take a moment for some deep breathing or a walk outside."

When your child follows expectations by carrying out the bedtime routine without protest, praise them and acknowledge their efforts to change their behavior. Give them the same amount of or more attention for their positive behaviors as the negative attention they would have received for their misbehaviors. Lastly, of course, follow through on delivering the agreed-upon reward.

Vignette: The Demander

Sonia and Barry have a ten-year-old son, Mateo, who ignores his parents' call to get ready for bed, and on the second or third reminder, he either says "five more minutes" or protests altogether ("No, I don't want to!"). That's when Sonia and Barry's eyes meet, each hoping the other will be the one to persuade Mateo to get ready for bed. Last week, Sonia went up to Mateo's room at bedtime and found him playing with toys on the floor. When Sonia began to direct him to clean up, he threw a toy at her! She directed him to retrieve it and put it away. She remained frustrated that he always seemed to behave like this at bedtime. She and Barry were beyond ready to make necessary changes to Mateo's bedtime routine.

With the guidance of Banish Bedtime Battles, *Sonia and Barry recognize the challenging behavior of their son in The Demander. They raise the subject of the new bedtime plan with Mateo.*

> *Sonia to Mateo: "Bedtime has been pretty tough for you lately, hasn't it?"*
>
> *Mateo: "Huh?"*
>
> *Sonia: "I mean that you seem to have a hard time following directions and keeping a calm body when it's time for bed."*
>
> *Mateo: "Yeah, I guess, but only because you won't let me stay up."*
>
> *Barry: "Your mom and I have been thinking about how to make it easier for you to get ready for bed."*

Mateo: *"How would you do that?"*

Sonia: *"Glad you asked! Well, we came up with a way to reward you for following bedtime expectations."*

Mateo: *"Cool! Reward me with what?"*

Barry: *"That's something we need you to help us figure out!"*

Mateo: *"Okay . . . "*

Sonia: *"Your Dad and I expect you to get ready for bed when we tell you to without any extra reminders or arguing. Is that something you can do?"*

Mateo: *"Yeah, I think so. It's just so hard because bedtime is so boring."*

Sonia: *"Bedtime IS quiet, and it's supposed to be relaxing, so I can see why you would find it boring. I wonder if there's a way to make up for that by doing something fun during the day."*

Sonia and Barry communicate their expectations for bedtime which involve getting ready for bed at 8:30 p.m. Sonia explains, "This means that at 8:30 p.m., you'll stop what you're doing, get changed, brush your teeth, wash your face, and get into your bed by 9:00 p.m. Then at 9:00 p.m., one of us will tuck you in. You may choose a book for reading or a relaxation exercise we can do together. This will be a lot different than you've been used to, but we can do it! Of course, we'll still be here to make sure you don't forget what's expected. Let's make a poster to remind us of what bedtime will be like so we can stay organized. Let's jot down what is expected at bedtime on a paper that you can put in your room. You can even list the reward you want to earn."

Then they establish Mateo's reward for following bedtime expectations on six out of seven nights—Mateo wants to earn an extra family game night this week.

On Sunday, the first night of the new routine, the family is relaxing in the living room and Mateo is watching his favorite TV show. Mateo's TV show ends at 8:30 p.m., signaling that it's time for his *bedtime routine to start. Barry says, "Okay, Mateo, time to get ready for bed. You've got this!" Mateo jumps up without hesitation and gets ready for bed as planned. His parents think, "That was easy!" They praise Mateo and reward him with one sticker for following the plan (five more to go to earn the reward this week).*

The next evening, however, when Sonia and Barry prompt Mateo to get ready for bed, Mateo requests to watch TV a little longer. Sonia responds warmly and firmly, "You really want to finish watching your movie tonight, but we're sticking to the bedtime plan."

Mateo begins whining and throws the remote control to the floor. Sonia recognizes that this may be an extinction burst (when child behavior gets worse once parents hold to a firm rule) and she is undeterred—she is committed to staying the course to let Mateo know, in no uncertain terms, that she will not bend on the rules. Sonia stands and nonverbally guides Mateo toward the bathroom. Mateo continues to complain. Sonia practices planned ignoring and maintains a nonverbal presence near the bathroom until Mateo has finished washing up and then guides him into bed. She says, "We had a little hiccup tonight, but this change in routine is still new so we have some kinks to work out. The good news is you can still earn your reward on Saturday if you earn a sticker every night for the rest of the week. Let's try again tomorrow." Mateo nods as he crawls in bed. Sonia models a mindful breathing exercise.

The Curtain Caller

After being tucked in for the night, my child calls out, gets out of bed multiple times with complaints and requests, makes a lot of noise, or joins me in my bed (with or without my knowledge) one or more times during the night.

Curtain calling is described here as a post-bedtime problem, but a Curtain Caller may also present with some pre-bedtime Demander characteristics. If this is the case for your child, you might consider a blend of the two plans.

Parents facing this battle will begin by supporting their child's use of coping strategies at bedtime. Clearly convey to your child that you have confidence in their ability to cope and that their bedroom is a safe place. Making your child go back to bed in the middle of the night is an opportunity to illustrate these two points. Middle-of-the-night returns to the bedroom should be completed in silence. In the morning, tell your child that you believe in their ability to cope with being alone in the dark, be explicit about their safety in their bedroom, and be warm and firm in conveying the expectation of remaining in their bed all night.

Building skills for emotional regulation is important because your child is seeking you out to help them regulate their emotions. Helping your child to manage their emotions is necessary from time to time; however, an overreliance on this parental help is detrimental to your child. If your child comes to rely solely on you for emotional regulation, they learn to seek you out every time they feel mildly uncomfortable, anxious, or distressed; hence, the curtain calls.

As your child learns to use emotion regulation strategies (e.g., mindful deep breathing, muscle relaxation, cognitive restructuring) more independently, you'll also want to use shaping to develop their staying-in-bed behavior. Shaping that stay-in-bed behavior looks like the following: tuck your child in, do mindful deep breathing or muscle relaxation, then explain, "If you remain quiet and in bed, I'm going to come back and check on you. If you call out, I will not return until you are quiet." Then, nonverbally check on them from the doorway after two minutes of silence to reinforce their quiet-staying-in-bed behavior. As they continue to follow your expectations, check on them again after five to ten minutes, but only if they remain quiet. Use planned ignoring if your child calls out and do not return for the check unless they have been quiet for a sustained period of time. Continue this method until your child is sleeping.

This "Quiet Check" method helps your child get used to remaining in their bed for longer and longer periods of time, and their efforts get positively reinforced by your nonverbal attention. Another approach for getting your child to sleep without you present is to gradually decrease the time spent in their presence and to gradually increase the physical distance between you and your child as they are tucked in and ready to sleep. See The Host for a full description of this procedure.

If your child does not stay in bed after bedtime, gesture or verbally redirect them back to bed. If possible, avoid walking them back to their room due to its reinforcing nature, and don't give them another tuck-in for the same reason. Remember to use planned ignoring as needed. Reward systems can be key in motivating your child to remain in their bed and quiet throughout the night.

Some reasons that children curtain call include fear of being alone in the dark, belief that they are missing out on post-bedtime fun, boredom, lack of sleepiness due to a bedtime that is too early, eating too much too late, and use of "screens" too close to bedtime. Consider the reason(s) your child is curtain calling. Figuring it out may take some detective work that involves talking with your child about the issue, using your own inductive reasoning skills, and a bit of trial and error. Take steps to solve any identified issues. For example, if you suspect your child's late-night snacking is disrupting their sleep, take steps to ensure an earlier snack time.

In short, solve what you can given what you've learned in Weeks 1–2. Lead your child through the coping skills in Week 3 until they can self-regulate and then positively reinforce your child's staying-quiet-and-in-bed behavior by checking on them only when they are quiet and in bed.

Make your bed uninviting to your child. While middle-of-the-night visitors are disruptive to your sleep, avoid the temptation to sleep elsewhere (e.g., couch) to get some sleep. When you or a bed partner sleep elsewhere, you are actually encouraging the unwanted behavior. Don't light the hallway to guide the middle-of-the-night trip, and eliminate extra pillows or other comforts in your bedroom that may attract your child.

If you are a parent who wakes in the morning surprised to find your child has sneaked into bed in the night, consider closing your bedroom door at night and placing a bell on the doorknob. Ensure that the lightest sleeper in your bed is closest to the bedroom door. If you sleep alone, position yourself on the bed in a fashion where you will awaken if your child slips into your bed.

Vignette: The Curtain Caller

Shea's nine-year-old son, Michael, is a Curtain Caller. Shea is diligently implementing the key parenting strategies in Banish Bedtime Battles *and has already adjusted Michael's bedtime based on what he's learned. Though Michael's bedtime routine is now more structured, Michael continues to curtain call after being tucked in for the night. Michael calls out "Dad . . . Dad . . . Dad?" until Shea goes into Michael's bedroom and gives him reassurance that there are no monsters in his closet. From monsters to burglars, noises, and strange lights on the ceiling, Michael finds something to be afraid of each night. Michael and Shea repeat the cycle of curtain calling and providing reassurance as many as three or four times in one night. Often, Shea just gives up and allows Michael into his bed.*

Shea is ready to banish this bedtime battle. Following the recommendations for The Curtain Caller, he raises the subject with Michael one morning at breakfast. Shea starts, "I've been thinking about how tough it is for you to sleep alone in your room . . . " Michael excitedly jumps in, "So do I get to sleep in your room now?" Shea smiles and says, "Not quite . . . I know you like having me close for comfort at night, but let's build your brave muscles and help you get more comfortable with sleeping independently," Michael's face falls. Michael says, "I don't know if I can." Shea says, "Well, I know you can. I know it sounds hard now but we're in this together."

Shea explains to Michael that he can earn a special outing with his best friend for his efforts in making the new bedtime plan work. Shea explains the new bedtime plan ("As long as you don't call out or get up after bedtime, except for emergencies, I'll come back in and check on you after a few minutes") and puts it into action that night.

Upon tucking Michael in, Shea leads Michael through a mindful breathing exercise and encourages Michael to practice it when he is feeling nervous in bed. Shea kisses Michael goodnight and says, "As long as you don't call out or get up now, I'll come back and check on you in a few minutes." Shea leaves Michael's bedroom, shuts the door behind him, and waits for two minutes to elapse on his watch. After two minutes, Shea returns to Michael's door, quietly opens it, and upon checking on Michael, he sees that Michael is staring back at him. Shea says, "I told you I'd be back. Great job being brave! Goodnight, Michael." Shea quietly shuts Michael's door and checks the time on his watch so he can return in five minutes. When five minutes have passed, Shea returns to Michael's bedroom and peers in to find Michael close to sleep. Shea smiles and shuts the door behind him.

Shea praises Michael in the morning for successfully falling asleep on his own. Shea keeps up the bedtime plan every night that week. Michael never called or got out of bed once! Shea follows through on the reward system he and Michael agreed upon earlier in the week and celebrates Michael's efforts to adapt to change.

The Ritualizer

My child obsesses over going to bed at a certain time and becomes anxious if they're "behind schedule," or they have difficulty falling asleep if certain bedtime conditions are not present (e.g., a certain movie playing, a song, or pillow arrangement).

It is probably not news to you that your child's insistence on a solid and unwavering routine is both a benefit and a limitation. Your child is highly predictable and may even be incredibly prompt. They crave routine and sameness. Life has a way of throwing us curve balls, however, which are not well tolerated by children who demand highly structured and unchanging routines. Thus, your child may fall to pieces when there is a small deviation from the expected or desired plan. Change *is* inevitable, and your child will benefit from being flexible and adaptable in response.

First, let's start with your child's distress over small deviations in their schedule. Our goal here is to demonstrate to your child that nothing "bad" happens if their schedule is changed, either intentionally or unintentionally. We want your child to become confident that they can manage the small to moderate amounts of distress or anxiety caused by unexpected or undesirable changes to their normal bedtime routine. While the focus here is on bedtime routines, keep in mind that the benefits to your child of increased flexibility and adaptability will extend to other daily routines and structured events as well.

Teach your child that spontaneity is desirable and can be loads of fun! If your child tends to view things that are new or unknown in a negative light, help them to see that, while they may be right some of the time, other times, they will be completely wrong. Remind them of times that they resisted something new (e.g., playing a new sport) only to discover that they loved it! Parents and children can have tons of fun testing out this new perspective—that change can not only be tolerated but also can be delightful and confidence-building. Your child cannot stop change from occurring, but they can learn to believe in their capacity to handle it when it does occur.

Assuming your child has a solid (maybe too solid) bedtime routine, build their tolerance for change and flexibility by varying it. Occasionally, you and your child can experiment by

- Starting the bedtime routine at the end (i.e., reverse the order of events).
- Starting the routine ten minutes early or ten minutes late.

- Doing elements of the bedtime routine out of order (e.g., brush teeth and then wash face instead of vice versa).

- Skipping a step in the routine (one night of going to bed with an unwashed face won't hurt anyone).

- Sleeping in regular clothes instead of pajamas (or wearing pajamas during part of the day!).

Extend this flexibility in routine to other areas of your child's day. Eat dessert first, drive home from dance lessons a different way than usual, have breakfast for dinner, go to the park in a neighboring town, eat hot dogs on hamburger buns and hamburgers on hot dog buns! Be playful and have fun with it! These flexibility-building capers will go a long way in helping your child to learn that novelty, spontaneity, and change can be fun.

Next, let's tackle the battle in which your child insists on using one or more items in their bedroom for the purpose of facilitating sleep. For example, you may have a child who insists on falling asleep to a particular movie each night. Or perhaps your child requires a certain placement of stuffed animals in the bedroom before they can fall asleep. The longer these routines go on, the stronger the sleep association and, you guessed it, the harder to undo!

When the pattern was first taking shape, you may have thought it harmless, even helpful or convenient. As time passes, however, you may question whether your view is correct, as your child is becoming increasingly rigid and demanding and less able to adapt to minor environmental or routine changes that may arise (e.g., vacations, room sharing). The general idea here is to gradually decrease the reliance on the object or situation that must be in place for sleep to occur (i.e., gradually undo the sleep association). For example, if your child insists on the placement of certain stuffed animals about the bed to fall asleep, try giving one animal a "sleepover" in another room of the home for a night or two, swap out one of the animals for a less preferred one, rearrange the position of the stuffed toys, or reduce the number of them gradually. Perhaps the stuffed animals are bored of their routine and are longing for an adventure, or perhaps the nighttime routine involves telling a story in which the stuffed animals are moved about the room and left in their places at the story's conclusion each evening. In sum, use a playful approach to build your child's enthusiasm for the plan.

Imagine another example in which a child is reliant upon a humming fan next to their bed to fall asleep. In this case, the fan might be moved farther and farther from the bed each night until it is no longer in the room. Alternatively, the fan might be replaced by a less desirable fan, a smaller/quieter fan, or run at a reduced speed. Or you might replace the fan with a sound machine (or virtual assistive technology such as Alexa) that produces a similar sound which can be lowered in volume across time until the sound is no longer required for sleep. Another option could be to drop the use of the preferred item (fan, in this case) altogether and go cold turkey. Cold turkey approaches tend to meet with success in shorter periods of time; however, they are often not well tolerated by children.

Vignette: The Ritualizer

Marin, the eleven-year-old daughter of Jade-Ann and Tyrone, has always been a child who prefers routine. She eats the same cereal for breakfast each day, insists on leaving for the school bus at 7:42 a.m. and not a minute earlier or later, and follows an after-school routine of her own making with the precision of an army sergeant. She becomes upset, tearful, and often angry when her routines are disrupted. Her night-time routine is no exception. Marin dictates her parents' and siblings' social schedules due to her insistence on being home before 8 p.m. so that she can start her bedtime routine on time.

Jade-Ann and Tyrone have grown concerned about Marin's rigid adherence to her routines. They miss the days when they could be spontaneous with her, and they worry about her ability to cope with the changes that inevitably occur in life. They think that Marin's rigidity, especially at bedtime, is limiting her confidence and skill in managing change and is putting a damper on her social life. Marin has been invited to vacations with cousins and sleepovers with friends but refuses to depart from her regular routines and, thus, turns down the offers. Also, Marin's insistence on routine has limited her parents' and siblings' opportunities to attend evening events, go on vacations and outings, and have guests in the home in the evenings. Jade-Ann and Tyrone recognize that Marin's behaviors are consistent with The Ritualizer, and they follow the recommendations associated with that bedtime battle.

Jade-Ann and Tyrone talk with Marin about their concerns, noting that Marin's preference for routine is both a help and a hindrance. They point out that routines are great for efficiency and predictability but not if one is unable to be flexible from time to time. In their effort to increase Marin's ability to be flexible at bedtime, they introduce the notion of "Flexible Fridays," during which they will have fun deviating from the normal bedtime routine and schedule. They enlist the help of Marin in brainstorming fun ways to be flexible on Fridays. The list they generated for the first Flexible Friday is below:

- *Eat a different snack (e.g., crackers and cheese) before bed instead of the usual one.*
- *Start the bedtime routine at 8:10 p.m. instead of 8:00 p.m.*
- *Wear a bathing suit to bed instead of pajamas (hey, we're having fun here!).*
- *Sleep backward on the bed (feet where the pillow usually is).*

Marin selects three of the new changes to implement on Friday. Following a successful and fun Flexible Friday, they add "Mix-It-Up Mondays" and "Wacky Wednesdays" to the weekly plan. Marin and her parents spend time each week thinking of ways to alter the nighttime routine while adhering to the basic start and end times (give or take fifteen minutes). Jade-Ann and Tyrone ask Marin how she's handling the changes, and Marin says that change was hard at first but it got easier. Jade-Ann points out that despite Marin's discomfort she handled the changes like a trooper! Marin concedes that she's had a lot of fun preparing for the new changes—she's spent more time with her parents and laughed a lot!

Her parents reward her efforts with praise, physical affection, and, in the spirit of enhanced flexibility, ice cream for breakfast one morning! Marin herself is delighted with the flexibility challenges and wants to extend them into her daytime routines. Jade-Ann and Tyrone get the whole family in on the action, seeking opportunities for spontaneity, embracing inevitable changes, and making sure to point out the good that has resulted from the expected (and unexpected) changes.

A Word about Night-Lights

It is common for children to rely on the use of night-lights and electronic devices to illuminate their bedroom at bedtime. For many of these children, they feel too afraid of the dark to go without them and want to avoid total darkness. The night-lights and electronic devices accommodate their fear, making it harder to overcome.

If your child uses night-lights or electronic devices, it is best to phase them out of the bedtime routine because doing so will ultimately make your child less fearful, build your child's confidence, and support healthy sleep. Make use of the Step-by-Step Transition Plan worksheet mentioned earlier in this week's reading to develop your plan to phase out the lights or electronic devices. You can access it at the end of this week's reading.

Because the phasing out process will no doubt be difficult, we suggest that you gradually, over nights (and maybe weeks), reduce the reliance on the lighting. For example, if your child demands the use of one or more night-lights, use a lower wattage bulb, decrease the number of lights in use, or increase the distance between the night-light and your child's bed.

Remember, human physiology calls for darkness for sleep. Our eyes need the nighttime sleep hours to rest. We do recognize and support, however, the use of night-lights for the purpose of illuminating a path through a dark room or hallway so that one can safely get from point A to B. When needed, use a soft light to illuminate the path.

THE SECRETS TO PUTTING IT ALL TOGETHER

In the following section, we will review the things you'll certainly want to do, as well as those you'll want to avoid as you transition to the new bedtime routine.

What to Do

1. Be calm, no matter how frustrated, angry, or exhausted you may be. Believe it or not, even negative communications and interactions can be rewarding to children, causing them to repeat the frustrating behaviors in the future.

2. If your child gets out of bed after their bedtime, you should, in as few words as possible, firmly direct them to return to their bed. If they do not respond to your verbal commands, you should nonverbally guide them back to bed. As tempting as it is, try to say as little as possible as you walk them back to their bedroom. And no matter how many times it takes (and we *really* mean this), guide your child back to bed. Two or two hundred times—nonverbally guide them back to their bed. This step is critical for the successful transition to independent sleeping.

3. Cuddling with your child at nighttime is one of the greatest pleasures of parenting. If you are concerned that your snuggling will interfere with the process of your child going to sleep independently (e.g., your child often falls asleep during

cuddling—or you do!), then you'll want to do it differently. We will *never* ask you to eliminate this bonding time, but we will ask you to move it to a different place. For example, you can keep the snuggles out of your child's bed and do it elsewhere, like in a comfy chair or another quiet place. You can also do it at a different time, like at the beginning of the routine or even just prior to the beginning of the routine.

4. This week, you will find thousands of opportunities to practice being warm and firm (Balanced parenting). You can be warm and firm regarding when homework is done, whether your child's room is cleaned, how much time is spent playing video games, and when the chores need to be done. A warm and firm parenting approach isn't just limited to enforcing the rules or correcting negative behaviors; it can be used to support positive behaviors as well! You can also be warm and firm when requiring that the family spends time together on the weekend, when your child receives praise and compliments for a job well done, and when family members engage in behaviors that reflect your family's values.

    For some parents, a reliance on this warm and firm approach will be an important shift in your parenting that is likely to have many long-term benefits. Your child will feel supported and will, over time, reduce unruly behaviors and increase the type of behavior you wish to see.

5. You'll need to distinguish between when your child is asking questions to obtain information (e.g., "What time will you be picking me up from my friend's house?" or "How old is Grandpa?") versus questions designed to elicit reassurance from you (e.g., "Will you be picking me up from my friend's house? Are you sure you will be there? What time are you going to get there?"). You are encouraged to answer the former but try to avoid too much conversation around the latter.

If your child seeks reassurance, say in a sincere and thoughtful manner: "What would you say?" or "What do you think?" or "What has happened in the past?" Refusing to answer such questions by flipping the question back to your child, helps them, first, to begin to tolerate mild discomfort associated with not having an immediate answer, and second, to trust their own judgment and thought processes. Asking your child to answer their own questions encourages them to become an independent thinker—a critical life skill!

6. Build, support, and strengthen calming and coping skills. Remember to reinforce mindful breathing and relaxation skills. Feel free to practice these right along with your child! Doing so will help your child remember to use the skills, see that you, too, believe in them, and normalize their use. On a related note, it is critical that you, as a parent, remain as calm as possible during this transition period. Your child, as always, will follow your lead. Calm begets calm. If you are at your wits' end during an unanticipated bedtime battle, call in the reserves (if you have them), and if not, take a break and come back to it when you have regrouped and composed yourself.

7. Use the process of shaping to achieve desired behaviors and use rewards to cement those gains. Recall that shaping is a process that involves teaching a child one new skill at a time. Each new skill is reinforced before another new skill is added. So if you want your child to follow the new bedtime routine, first, make sure that they are familiar with it and reward them if they can repeat it. Next, praise them for completing the first step of the routine (say, toothbrushing). Once they reliably start the bedtime routine with toothbrushing, add in the next step, say, face washing. Now your child is only praised after completion of both behaviors. Then, add the third step, pajamas! Now your child is praised

only after teeth are brushed, face is washed, and pajamas are on. You get the picture. This shaping procedure is incredibly useful in teaching a wide variety of desired behaviors to your child and other family members!

8. During the transition to independent sleeping, you *will* lose sleep. You *will* be tired. You *will* have doubts about whether you are doing things right. Reach out to others and let them know that you have begun this process. Accept help if offered. Give yourself a little more forgiveness than you ordinarily do. This period is a tough one, but don't lose sight of the benefits that lie ahead. Short-term sleep loss is traded for long-term sleep-filled blissful nights! But to get there, you need to ensure that you are at your best. Be sure to engage in those activities you know help to rejuvenate you and restore your energy when you are run-down—exercise, time outdoors, solitude, baking, helping a friend, journaling, reading, meditating, volunteering, connecting with a friend—find and do the activities that fortify you.

What Not to Do

1. Do not lock doors (yours or your child's), shame or embarrass your child if they get out of their bed, yell, or punish your child. When positive praise and small rewards are used along with clear expectations and limits, there is usually no need for punishment. There is plenty of research evidence documenting that punishment is less effective than the application of positives when attempting to change child behaviors.[1] Punishments may seem to work in the short-term, but they do not promote lasting change and may increase the risk of your child engaging in physical or verbal aggression in the future.[2]

2. Avoid "magical solutions" such as sleep fairy dust, anti-monster spray, or other potions and lotions. These

so-called solutions to sleep problems do not permit your child to take the credit for their sleeping progress. If your child manages to stay in bed all night, they are apt to credit the "potion" with their success rather than their own efforts. In such a case, the child learns that their successes are produced or determined by external factors rather than internal ones (such as grit, motivation, persistence, and effort). We want your child to learn the direct connection between their hard work and their successes.

3. Refrain from the use of "safety" behaviors. Safety behaviors are those that are completed to make one feel more comfortable or to prevent a feared event from happening. "So, what's so bad about that?" you ask. Good question! Safety behaviors (e.g., looking both ways when crossing a road) can be necessary when used in the face of a real threat to one's well-being (e.g., getting hit by a car). When a safety behavior is used in an anxiety-provoking but safe situation (e.g., lying in bed alone at night), however, its use can prevent the child from learning that their fear is unwarranted. For example, using additional lighting in your child's bedroom at night (a safety behavior) serves to validate your child's fear (the dark is scary), undermines their self-competence (they believe they can't handle being in the dark), and prevents your child from learning over time that their feared scenario does not come to pass (no monster comes out from under the bed in the dark). Safety behaviors, a form of accommodation, prevent your child from learning from the experience of facing their fears.

4. Avoid the temptation to lay with your child until they fall asleep or to sleep with them or near to them unless it is a part of your plan to reshape your child's bedtime behavior. If you find yourself craving the closeness of your child, just move this important cuddling time to a different time

during the day. Again, we'll never ask you to eliminate this critical connection with your child, but we will ask you to move it to a time that allows for a successful bedtime routine. It is critically important that your child develops the skill of falling asleep on their own, without your presence. This skill paves the way for your child to fall back to sleep after middle-of-the-night awakenings, makes sleepovers with family or friends possible for your child, and permits you to engage in some overnight travel without your child.

5. Limit discussions of the bedtime routine or changes to the routine, avoid debates about the routine, and refrain from persuasive tactics (yours or your child's) at night. Keep these types of discussions to daytime hours. If it's helpful, you and your child can keep a list of the discussion points as they arise, but do not discuss them until morning. At night, you and your child are likely tired, and things often seem worse, more negative, or, well, just darker at night. Additionally, these kinds of discussions can be quite stimulating, thus getting in the way of sleep. Trust us, do not debate or discuss after dark!

6. Avoid offering excessive reassurance. Refer to point number 5 in the What to Do section above to help you distinguish between requests for information and requests for reassurance. When you provide excessive reassurance to your child (and we know the temptation is great), you increase the likelihood of your child asking for help and reassurance again in the future, you send a subtle message that they are unable to cope and think on their own, you validate their fears and anxiety, and you unwittingly send a vote of no confidence. No parent wants to do that!

7. Don't give up or give in! Okay, we know this is easier said than done, but you've got the knowledge and the motivation,

or you wouldn't have gotten this far. So, stay the course! You are on the verge of a whole new way of living—with sleep and without bedtime battles! Ensure that you are getting the self-care and support you need so that you have the energy and resources to sustain the course.

One final note, we often hear from children and parents about the imagined dreadful consequences of lost sleep. We hear irrational beliefs about a night or two of imperfect sleep both from children who fear being unable to sleep without a parent or loved one close by *and* from parents who worry about possible negative effects of lost sleep, like distraction at school, poor grades, subpar performance at sports or other extracurricular activities. A common belief about sleep loss includes, "If my child doesn't get a full night's sleep, they'll have a horrible day tomorrow." It is important to challenge this belief and similar ones. While it's no fun to slog through the day after a night of poor sleep, there are no real catastrophic consequences of doing so. In fact, most Americans do it. While we don't want you or your child to join that group, we want to emphasize that imagined calamitous outcomes from one night of poor sleep are greatly overblown. Tired? Yes. Tragedy? No.

 Now Apply It!

It's go time! Implement your child's new bedtime plan based on the recommendations for your specific battle type. Remember that the rollout of the plan should be clear to your child and gradual in nature. The Step-by-Step Transition Plan worksheet* will be helpful in ensuring that the changes are made at a reasonable pace for your child. Check back to the Ideal Bedtime Routine worksheet* from Week 1 to be sure that you haven't forgotten anything you had originally planned.

---

*Access the worksheets by scanning the QR code below or by going to www.highperformance-parenting .com/bbb-appendices.

WEEK 5 SUMMARY

- Week 5 is about making big changes at bedtime. Decide whether you want to use a gradual approach to change (recommended) or an all-at-once approach.

- Remember to keep the bedtime routine to thirty minutes, limit technology use in the hour leading up to bedtime, be aware of sleep associations, limit caffeine intake and other sleep-hindering eating habits, and use Balanced parenting (be warm and firm!).

- Implement your new bedtime plan.
  - The Host: The child who sleeps only if a parent lies with them in their bed until they fall asleep *or* if a parent is near them as they go to sleep.
    - Gradually, decrease time spent together at bedtime and increase distance between child and parent as the child falls asleep.
  - The Roommate: The child who sleeps only if they lie with a parent in the parent's bed until they fall asleep *or* if a parent is near them as they go to sleep.
    - Shift the child's sleep location to their bed, decrease time spent together at bedtime, and

increase distance between child and parent as the child falls asleep.

- ° The Bed Warmer: The child who falls asleep only in the parent's bed and can do so independently.

    - ♦ Shift the child's sleep location to their own bed either gradually or all in one night.

- ° The Demander: My child protests or has tantrums when told to begin their bedtime routine or to get into bed.

    - ♦ Help the child learn to independently manage their distress and control their emotions using mindful deep breathing and relaxation skills. Set and enforce compliance with family expectations for bedtime. Reward successes.

- ° The Curtain Caller: The child who calls out for parents, gets out of bed multiple times, or joins parents in their bed (with or without parent's knowledge) one or more times during the night.

    - ♦ Teach the child coping strategies to use independently when distressed, motivate the child with rewards to remain in bed, use planned ignoring, and consistently return the child back to bed with little to no talking.

- ° The Ritualizer: The child who obsesses over going to bed at a certain time and becomes anxious if they're "behind schedule" or has difficulty falling asleep if certain bedtime conditions are not present.

    - ♦ Decrease the child's reliance on the objects they require for sleep, increase the child's flexibility, and adjust the child's beliefs about change.

- • Many children rely on night-lights to help them to feel more comfortable at night. Yet night-lights accommodate fear and can actually increase the fear over time. If your child uses night-lights, phase them out over time to decrease your child's fear and build their confidence.

- What to do as you implement the new sleep plan:
  - Stay calm. Your child wants attention, even if it may be negative.
  - Consistently and quietly redirect your child back to their bed each time they get out.
  - Move parent-child togetherness to an earlier time and a place other than your child's bed.
  - Practice being warm and firm at bedtime as well as throughout the day.
  - Distinguish between questions about necessary information or facts versus questions designed to elicit reassurance from you. Answer the former. Ignore the latter.
  - Build your child's coping skills through repeated practice.
  - Use shaping to achieve desired behaviors, and use rewards to cement those gains.
  - Don't forget to take care of yourself. This will be hard work.
- What *not* to do as you implement the new sleep plan:
  - Do not lock bedroom doors, shame, embarrass, or punish your child if they get out of their bed or call out.
  - Avoid "magical" sleep solutions that allow your child to credit the "potion" with their success rather than their own efforts.
  - Refrain from use of "safety" behaviors, which serve to accommodate fears.

- Do not lie with your child until they fall asleep. Leave the room before they fall asleep.

- Limit nighttime discussions of the bedtime routines or changes to the routine. Hold these conversations during the day.

- Avoid providing excessive reassurance to your child.

- Don't give up or give in! Commit to the bedtime plan and stay the course.

Battle No More

CONGRATULATIONS! YOU DID IT. WHEW, THE WORST IS LIKELY over. It is now essential to maintain the changes that you have made. Your child's new behaviors are not yet deep set so continue to stick firmly to the new bedtime routine and sleeping arrangements. Bedtime battles, if they remain present at this time, will continue to lessen, and eventually disappear so long as you hold fast to the plan that you have created to ensure your child's best sleeping habits. Consistency is key!

There will come a time when you can be more flexible with the nighttime routine, but you aren't there yet. Give the new routine a couple of months before you decide to change something, and when you do, keep those changes to one night only. Ensure that the changes are infrequent, short-lived (no more than a night or two), and clearly communicated to your child as temporary changes.

MAINTENANCE OF INDEPENDENT SLEEP

Be consistent. Because consistency is the key to sustainable change, it is paramount not only that you enforce the bedtime routine each night but also that you ensure that other key people in your child's life are knowledgeable and hold fast to the bedtime routine as well. If your child has regular visits with an ex-partner, grandparents, other relatives, or friends, take the time to explain to them the hard work that you've done to help your child become an independent sleeper, and ask them to honor your efforts by requiring your child to follow a similar routine at their home. We want your child to see healthy nighttime habits as behaviors that are important in their own right and not as behaviors that are dependent upon the setting. For example, we want your child to believe that they engage in a nighttime routine because it is good for them, and not because they are at a particular location (e.g., at home).

Use praise. It is important to positively reinforce your child's increased independence with praise. Some parents mistakenly believe that they need to praise their child only when attempting to initiate a new pattern of behavior. Not so! It is critical to keep the praise coming, though over time, you can make it more intermittent and less expected. Intermittent or sporadic praise often leads the child to engage in the desired behavior at very high rates in efforts to achieve that parental praise!

The wording of your praise matters too. One type of meaningful praise places a focus on effort. Praising your child's effort on a particular task ("You worked really hard on that homework!") results in children who approach challenges and see their efforts as instrumental in reaching their goals. A second type of meaningful praise involves praising a trait or ability ("Wow, you're a great artist!"). This type teaches children that what is valuable is the individual characteristic or ability of the child. These two types of praise teach children different reasons for their success (effort vs. trait). Acknowledging your child's positive behaviors can encourage continued independence and reduce a child's attempts to get more attention through less desirable behaviors. Praise the behaviors you like, and you'll see more of them. It's an age-old, fool-proof method for changing your child's behaviors for the better.

Practice calming skills. Encourage your child to continue the practice of mindful breathing and relaxation. Set some time aside each day to practice these skills. Initially, help your child to structure their day to include this practice, and practice right along with them. It will help you too! Then, after a few weeks, begin to encourage your child to practice these calming strategies independently as this will ensure that they can do it wherever and whenever they need it. Remember to keep up your encouragement! Your praise and support will be a powerful incentive for your child to continue the practice.

Show interest in your child's experiences with independent sleep. Talk to your child about how things are going as they master the new skill of independent sleeping. Ask them, "What's harder than you thought? What's easier than you thought?" Using this information, tweak the bedtime routine and sleeping environment as necessary, taking care to not indulge your child's fears or dislike of change. It's okay to compromise when doing so does not allow your child to break the established bedtime routine. For example, if your child wants to change the order of some of the steps in the bedtime routine, that's fine. However, if your child wants to avoid some steps or change the routine in a manner inconsistent with the goal of independent sleeping or that gives your child too much control in decision-making regarding the routine, use great caution before agreeing to the compromise.

Though you should remain warm and firm in your conversations about how your child's new sleep routine is going, do listen carefully and take seriously your child's fears, worries, and any misconceptions they may have about the new bedtime routine. Address fears and worries with care and concern. Help your child to think rationally about whether their fears are real or baseless (e.g., weigh the evidence for and against your child's worry—is the feared event likely or unlikely to occur?). If your child has misconceptions or misunderstandings about the new routine, ensure that your child has the correct information. For example, if your child believes that it is unfair for them to start their bedtime routine at 8 p.m. while an older sibling can stay up until 9 p.m., talk openly and clearly about the rights, responsibilities, and privileges that come with growing up. Whatever the misconception, endeavor to clear it up. Take the time needed to explain yourself, your intentions, the rules, and the gains that you expect will come from your actions and decisions.

Make a habit of checking in with your child about how they are handling new experiences, whether regarding sleeping or something else. Doing this sends your child the message that their daily experiences (including both struggles and successes) are important conversation topics for parents and children.

Promote a sense of self-competence. You and your child have accomplished something monumental. You set your sights on changing a behavior, and you have done it! Don't let the significance of this be lost on you or your child. Millions of people attempt to modify their behavior every day (e.g., more exercise, less junk food, no smoking, etc.), and these changes are difficult to achieve! Please note that the steps to change your child's bedtime behavior are the same general steps to change any behavior—define the change you want to see, commit to the change, reward behaviors that are closer and closer to the desired behavior, and ensure the new behavior is firmly entrenched before introducing flexibility or changes.

Help your child to see their amazing achievement! Promote their sense of competence by pointing out how they have used these general behavior-change skills in the past (e.g., learning to ride a bike, learning to read) and discuss that they will use these skills to make strides in the future. Children who believe that they can (1) set and reach goals and (2) face and overcome challenges are children who trust in their own ability to make positive changes around them. Look out world!

Celebrate with your child. As noted previously, your child has accomplished something big. Find ways to celebrate their achievement. Get others (e.g., siblings, grandparents, etc.) in on it. Celebrations create memorable marks in time that serve to solidify gains. While there are thousands of ways to celebrate your child's achievement, one of the most creative that we've come across is the use of a "celebration" dinner plate. The plate can be decorated at a paint-your-own pottery location or can simply be a plate that is denoted as special because it is *only* used by a family member or dinner guest who is celebrating an achievement. Again, get creative. Ellen has a family celebratory tradition in which family members do the "dance of joy" (a silly type of square dancing to a playful tune sung by family members) to commemorate a special event. The dance is a merry event that never gets old. Find your family's celebratory style and create a new tradition! We've included a certificate to get the party started! You can access it at the end of this week's reading.

TROUBLESHOOTING
There are few behavioral changes that occur smoothly and without the occasional setback. It is important, as you support your child in their independent sleeping, to have realistic expectations about how things will go. Let's face it—life happens. There will be illnesses, vacations, and disruptions of all sorts that may set you or your child off track. It is important to ensure that, as you assess your child's progress across time, you look at the changes in their behavior across weeks and months, and not across days. The real trajectory of behavior change is up and down from day-to-day but an upward slope over the course of weeks and months.

Below are some of the most common trouble spots and recommendations for how to handle them.

You sleep through it when your child crawls into bed with you in the middle of the night.

It's bound to happen. You wake in the morning after what you thought was a blissful night of sleep only to find that you have an interloper in your bed! No matter the time, gently wake and walk your child back to their bed. Do not chastise, yell, complain, or otherwise comment on the event. Later, when you are both fully awake and calm, reiterate the bedtime rule of staying in one's bed at night. Find out your child's thinking at the time and problem-solve solutions to help your child be successful in remaining in bed when they awaken at night.

If the behavior persists, consider the implementation of a reward system for nights that your child remains in their bed until wake-up time. It is most often the case that undesirable behaviors can be changed by rewarding their absence (child remains in bed all night and is rewarded with favorite breakfast in the morning), rather than by punishing their presence (child gets out of bed at night and has a consequence of no video games the following day). For additional strategies, refer to the Curtain Caller section of Week 5.

In a weak middle-of-the-night moment, you give in.

We can't always be at our best, especially when we are overtired and sleep deprived. If you find that, at your wits' end, you give in and allow your child to join you in bed or you join them in theirs, have confidence that not all is lost. Sticking with the bedtime plan on subsequent nights is all that is needed to correct the course. Let your child know that in a sleep-addled moment, you made an unwise choice. Model for your child how to admit a mistake and move forward with greater commitment to be consistent.

Your child's outbursts, tantrums, or crying worsen over time rather than go away.

When parents begin using a consistent approach to bedtime, ensuring that the nighttime routine is completed every night and holding firm to the independent sleeping plan, some children may show some undesirable behaviors. Because their tantrums, distress, whining, or other negative behaviors may have resulted in getting what they wanted in the past (e.g., parents ultimately let them sleep in the parents' bed), they will use these behaviors again in attempts to achieve the same result. When the parent remains firm, the child often escalates the behaviors (e.g., whining more, crying louder and longer) to achieve the result that these behaviors brought about in the past. They will whine, complain, and persist longer and harder, but thankfully, only to a point—the point at which they realize that these behaviors are not bringing about their end goal. At this point, the behaviors come to an end. During this process, however, many parents give up when the child's undesirable behaviors increase, assuming the plan isn't working. Rest assured, though, if this happens, it is a sign that you are on the right track! Stay the course.

Your child says some things that are upsetting, scary, and concerning to you.

We would be remiss if we did not acknowledge the possibility that your child may say or do some concerning things as they attempt to change your mind about sticking to the bedtime routine. Your child may threaten scary behaviors (e.g., running away, wanting to "die"). This is downright frightening for a parent. If your child makes threatening statements in the heat of the moment, be sure to discuss these statements at a time that you and your child are calm and collected. Ask your child about the statements they made. Determine if they feel this way at other times (outside of being asked to complete the nighttime routine). If so, how often do these thoughts occur? How long do they last? If your child lets you know that they have these feelings, impulses, or urges (e.g., to run away, to "die") at times other than when you asked them to modify their behavior, then it is a very good idea to seek out the help of a mental health professional. Ask your child to tell you if, when, and how often the thoughts occur. Together, determine a way for them to inform you when they have these thoughts (e.g., what language or phrasing can they use to let you know?).

If your child acknowledges that they did not really intend the threatening behavior and would never engage in such, help them to identify alternative means for trying to influence parent behavior. As one example of an alternative strategy, a child might be given the opportunity to thoughtfully and clearly "make their case" before a parent chooses how to respond. This strategy teaches your child many important lessons: they get practice in constructing a clear and compelling argument, they learn that you listen and take seriously their thoughts and opinions (though ultimately you may not give in to what they want), and you gain valuable information about your child's experiences that can help you to better assist your child in problem-solving difficult situations.

You've been using a reward system for more than a week without any real progress toward the bedtime plan.

It's time to do some problem-solving. One reason for the lack of progress may be that you have selected an ineffective reward. Remember that the only way to know if a reward is rewarding to your child is to hear it from them! To determine this, look to rewards that have worked in the past to change your child's behavior or simply ask your child what they might be willing to work toward. Be sure the rewards that they offer up are reasonable—we aren't talking about trips to Disney World here.

Relatedly, the selected reward may be less rewarding than the attention your child is getting from you for their bedtime battles. Remember that negative attention is often more valued than no attention. We also want to caution against switching to rewards of higher value as this may lead your child to learn to "hold out" for more extravagant rewards.

If rewards don't seem to be the issue for the lack of progress, you may also consider whether the required behavior is clear to your child and whether your child is *able* to perform the behavior you've asked for. Clarify, if the former, and scale back what is required for the latter.

Your child absolutely refuses to engage in the relaxation exercises or other strategies due to outright defiance or fear that they will eventually have to sleep alone.

Some headstrong children may refuse to engage in any of the strategies or behaviors designed to reduce fear and promote compliance with the nighttime routine. The good news is that parents have a lot of influence over child behaviors. As parents, how you respond to your child's behaviors will determine whether these behaviors increase or decrease across time. As such, your child is not solely responsible for the success of independent sleeping. Your parenting responses are most important! So if you continue to insist that your child remains in their bed at night, even the most stubborn or defiant child will eventually sleep independently when the parents provide a warm ("You can do it! We believe in you!") and firm ("We believe that it is best for you to sleep in your own bed each and every night, and we will not bend on this rule.") response.

Your child shares the details of their day with you only at bedtime, and you don't want to miss out on the valuable information.

We don't want you to miss those details either! We've found that sometimes children are more willing to talk at bedtime because they aren't directly face-to-face with a parent. If your child seems to open up only when you are lying side-by-side, try to find some time during the day to chat when you aren't face-to-face. Car rides and walks are perfect options for this. Or perhaps it's the physical closeness that gets your child talking. Try to sit close on the couch and see if that gets the conversation started. Sometimes parents need to experiment a little to find the conditions during which your child feels most comfortable to reveal their inner thoughts and feelings.

Your child struggles to sleep at friends' or relatives' homes.

Once your child has been consistently sleeping independently at home, it's time to start expanding the range of environments in which your child sleeps independently. Remember to start small. For example, you might wish to begin with a sleepover in the guest bedroom or your backyard. Alternatively, you might begin with a sleepover at Grandma's when parents are also staying so you are nearby but your child is sleeping independently in a new environment. Then, you may wish to progress to a stay at Grandma's without parents before moving on to a sleepover at a friend's home, for example.

It's a great idea to get your child's buy-in on the sleepover. Try to begin when they feel *almost* ready. Keep in mind that they won't feel *completely* ready until they've gone on ten or more sleepovers! Start with some brainstorming with them about how to make the sleepover more comfortable even if it will still be a little challenging for them. Remember that children learn how to handle challenging situations by handling challenging situations.

It is always important to involve your child in discussions about what is easier and harder for them. Decide how you will expand the places where your child can sleep with their input as your child is the only one who really knows what makes the experience difficult for them, though some children may have a difficult time expressing or even understanding the source of their fears or concerns. In this case, be an observant parent. Pay attention to the situations in which your child has a harder or easier time and gradually build up to more difficult sleeping environments.

Your child has anxiety about being away from you, both during the day and at night, making bedtimes very difficult.

A child who experiences separation anxiety is one who worries that something bad might happen to them or to their parents such that they would no longer be able to be together again. Separation anxiety often shows up at bedtime when children refuse to sleep without the presence of a parent. To help your child manage their anxiety, be sure to instill confidence in them. Let them know that they are safe and perfectly capable of managing themselves without you. Then, gradually require your child to spend longer and longer periods of time away from you and on their own. This will build their confidence and help to promote their coping skills.

Your child feels scared and worried as they lay down at night, making falling asleep difficult.

It's not uncommon for children to be scared at night. Worries and fears always loom larger as the day progresses to evening. Every thump becomes a burglar breaking in, every creak is a monster in the closet. While it will be tempting for you to reassure your child by locking the doors and windows each night or checking the closets for goblins, these strategies often backfire. Reassuring your child with your words or behaviors can send the message that your child's fears are legitimate. You *do* need to check the closet because there *could be* a monster inside. Refusing to indulge the fear will demonstrate that you believe that the child is perfectly safe to be alone in their bedroom at night.

During the day, your child's mind is distracted by a multitude of activities from classes and friends to extracurricular activities and homework. Once in bed for the night, their minds are free to dwell on past or present distressing situations (rumination) as well as worries about the future (anticipatory anxiety). These thoughts can cause their bodies to become more alert, raising heart rate, quickening breathing, and tensing muscles. Encourage your child to do some mindful breathing or relaxation exercises as discussed in Week 3. The focus on these activities will help to leave little to no room for the worried thoughts. These coping strategies also signal the brain that there is no imminent danger, allowing the body to settle and sleep to take over.

Another helpful strategy involves the use of a worry journal that is completed during the day. If your child gets the worried thoughts out of their head and onto paper, they are more likely to be able to empty their mind of the repetitive and distressing thoughts. Similarly, setting a fifteen-minute "worry time" during which your child can engage all those anxiety-provoking thoughts can help to reduce worries at nighttime. Just be sure that the time is set early in the day. Sometimes seeing anxious thoughts in print can help to shrink the worries down to size, help to identify potential solutions to problems, or lead to greater acceptance of the circumstances that can't be changed.

Your child takes a one- to two-hour nap each day after school and then has difficulty sleeping at night.

While naps can be a great way to catch up on lost sleep, routinely taking naps can interfere with the ability to fall asleep at night. Naps should be relatively brief (twenty to forty minutes). Napping longer than forty minutes allows you to go into the deeper stages of sleep because your brain thinks you are in for a full night. Then, when you wake from your nap, you may feel very groggy and sleepy just as you would if you were to get up in the middle of the night.

Your child insists on keeping their phone in their bedroom.

A family charging station where all phones "reside" at night is a good solution to this problem. Many children will dream up all sorts of reasons why they need their phones in their bedrooms at night. Listen and consider their grounds. If your child has a reasonable justification, and they can demonstrate responsible use for a sustained period, perhaps the phone can stay in the bedroom—far away from the bed. However, phones are best kept out of the bedroom at night—including yours.

Your child has nightmares that leave them feeling terrified to go to sleep each night.

No doubt about it, nightmares are pretty darn scary. Every child has a bad dream now and again. It's completely normal and expected. When your child wakes from a nightmare in the middle of the night, offer them acknowledgment of how frightening a bad dream can be. Your empathy will go a long way here. Be sure your child has mastered independent use of the deep breathing and relaxation strategies covered in this book. Those coping strategies will help to turn off the "fight-or-flight" arousal response that was set into motion by the nightmare. Ultimately, we want your child to learn how to settle themselves so that they are able to put themselves back to sleep.

Avoid the temptation to remove "scary" objects (e.g., dolls) from the room as doing so will inadvertently send your child the message that the dolls really *are* scary. Instead, encourage your child to gradually spend time with the feared object (or similar objects) so that they can learn that it is not as scary as they made it out to be in their mind.

Encouraging your child to come up with a new ending to the nightmare can be empowering, particularly if your child is victorious over the scary figure(s) in the revised ending. Encourage humorous endings (not violent) as humor and fear are a bit incompatible. If you are laughing, it's hard to be scared at the same time.

If your child is experiencing repeated nightmares that have begun to affect their functioning during the day as well as at bedtime, it's time to consult with your child's doctor.

You, as a parent, miss the nighttime togetherness that you shared prior to the new bedtime plan.

We hear you on this one! There is nothing better than the wonderful feelings brought about by closeness with your child. Don't forgo it at bedtime without replacing that physical closeness and conversation by doing it at another time and place. Many parents often ask if it is ever okay to sleep together after independent sleeping has begun. It is okay to sleep together occasionally *after* independent sleep is well established. Be absolutely sure that your child understands that this is a rare and special circumstance and a return to independent sleeping in their own bed will occur the following night.

You question whether you are doing the right thing.

Parenting is no easy feat, and all parents question themselves from time to time. It can feel wrong to lead a crying and distressed child back to their bedroom to sleep alone. A short-term solution is certainly to allow them into your bed or to sleep in theirs. This short-term solution, however, is short-sighted. We encourage you to think long-term.

Children who learn to sleep independently learn to develop and rely on their own coping skills. Developing these skills at bedtime permits the use of them in other challenging situations and environments. Children who sleep independently learn that their parents believe in their capacity to manage themselves, even when they are distressed (but safe). When parents believe in children, children learn to believe in themselves. It is certainly true that life's challenges are inevitable, and requiring your child to sleep independently is one step toward teaching your child that you and they can believe in their ability to manage hard things. Remember that line used by our professional colleague who tells her young children, "We learn to do hard things by doing hard things."

You share custody of your child with a former partner and your child's bedtime routine is now different across homes.

It is certainly preferred for both parents to follow the same plan, but we recognize that it's not always possible. Children will quickly learn what is expected of them in each household and behave accordingly. So if you're wondering if it's worth it to implement the bedtime plan in your home even if it is not implemented in your former partner's home, yes, it's worth it! One parent can follow the plan and reap the benefits, and the other can continue whatever pattern of interaction has been established within that household. However, there is a good possibility that the child who has learned to sleep independently, and is confident and comfortable at bedtime, will improve their nighttime behaviors within the other household as well.

You wonder how to prevent the same problems from occurring with your other (perhaps younger) children.

The good news is that you now know the ropes! Keeping your other children from following the same path (to your bedroom in the middle of the night!) is in your wheelhouse. You are in a great position to weigh the pros and cons of permitting co-sleeping, and you know the efforts involved in transitioning from bed sharing to independent sleeping. In this book, you've learned principles and strategies to avoid nighttime battles and to pave the way for calm and confidence at bedtime. Deciding what is in your child's best interest and then warmly and firmly insisting upon that course of action is a recipe for great parenting. It may be of benefit to revisit parts of the book (or even the whole book) with your other children in mind. Each child is unique and will likely require a different bedtime plan. Additionally, now that you've learned many of the most effective parenting practices, you've got some new tools in the parenting tool kit; odds are, bedtime may go very differently with your younger children. You've got this!

REFLECTION

Congratulations to you and your child on your tremendous efforts to implement independent sleeping! Yahoo! We had every confidence that you and your child would meet with success. Be sure to recognize your child's perseverance and celebrate your shared hard work! Print out a certificate of achievement that you can share with your child to celebrate their success. You can access one at the end of this week's reading. Steep the giving of the certificate in ceremony for an accomplishment your child will remember.

Emphasize how your child's willingness to be a little uncomfortable in the short run has made them braver, more independent, and a better sleeper in the long run.

While this book was written for the sole purpose of helping families to transition children to sleeping independently, readers have also learned a good number of effective parenting strategies along the way. These research-supported methods will help you to become the parent you were always meant to be! They are skills that can be used across many different types of situations in which parents and children can find themselves. They are not limited to parenting at nighttime.

If your child has not yet mastered the skill of independent sleep, don't give up! Success still lies ahead. Take a short break, reread all the Weeks, and give it another go. Take care not to feel defeated or be critical of your child. You will be teaching your child an exceptionally important life skill when you refuse to give up and try the plan again!

 Now Apply It!

Fill out the certificate of achievement,* present it to your child, and place it in a prominent position within your home! Celebrate with your child.

*Access the certificate by scanning the QR code below or by going to www.highperformance-parenting.com/bbb -appendices.

WEEK 6 SUMMARY

- Consistency is key! Ensure that you remain consistent in your child's bedtime routine and make sure others around your child (e.g., parenting partners, grandparents, friends) do the same.

- Intermittent praise helps ensure that your child will keep doing the desired behavior.

- Celebrate your child's accomplishments (and your own!).

- Slowly introduce the bedtime routine in other contexts (e.g., a babysitter is in charge, a sleepover at a grandparent's or friend's home).

- Sometimes setbacks happen! Look at the big picture changes from week-to-week rather than being discouraged by day-to-day troubles.

- Setbacks can be corrected through renewed focus on commitment to the bedtime routine and praising the behaviors you want to see.

Now It's Your Turn!

WAIT . . . WE KNOW WHAT YOU ARE THINKING. YOU THOUGHT this was a six-week plan, right? Well, you didn't think you were getting away without us talking about *your* sleep, did you? Now that your child is well on their way to sleeping independently, it's time to turn our attention to *your* sleep. Your sleep is just as important as your child's. In truth, it may be *more* important. In the preflight safety instructions in an airplane, you are instructed to place the oxygen mask over your own face before assisting your child. Similarly, you need to ensure that you are well rested to be the best parent you can be for your child. Lack of sleep is associated with higher levels of stress and related problems such as anxiety and depression. As anyone with children knows, parenting is a hard job, and parenting on insufficient sleep is near impossible. When you take care of your sleep needs first, you have the energy and focus necessary to ensure that your child's sleep needs are met.

We don't mean to say that getting proper sleep during parenthood is easy. It's not. A 2019 study published in the journal *Sleep* found that parents, especially mothers, continue to experience sleep loss and reduced sleep satisfaction for up to six years following the birth of their first child![1] Parenting, rife with innumerable rewards, certainly takes a toll on parent sleep.

The average adult needs at least seven hours of sleep each night, but research demonstrates that 35 percent of adults get fewer than seven hours.[2] Sleep insufficiency is so widespread that the U.S. Centers for Disease Control and Prevention (CDC) has declared insufficient sleep a "public health problem."

Why is sleep so hard to come by? It may be factors associated with our modern style of living, including everyday stressors (e.g., work demands, urban commuting, family struggles), excessive use of technology, nicotine and alcohol use, physical inactivity, and high-fat, high-sugar diets. These factors are all known to cause disruption in sleep.

In U.S. culture, sleep deprivation often seems to earn a badge of honor. Many U.S. leaders and business gurus glorify sleep deprivation. Former president Barack Obama reportedly slept five to six hours per night while in office.[3] Elon Musk too is said to come in at about six hours per night.[4] Former president Donald Trump has said that he sleeps about four hours per night, suggesting that one shouldn't sleep any more than they have to. He's even gone so far as to say, "I have friends who are successful and sleep ten hours a night, and I ask them, 'How can you compete against people like me if I sleep only four hours?' It rarely can be done. No matter how brilliant you are, there's not enough time in the day."[5] Despite what powerful people may say, sleep is a basic need, and sleep deprivation in adults comes with high personal and societal costs.

THE COSTS OF INSUFFICIENT SLEEP
A good night's sleep is critical to mental health and emotional well-being. The phrase "woke up on the wrong side of the bed" alludes to the fact that sleep can negatively affect one's mood and emotional functioning. The relationship between sleep and emotional functioning is bidirectional—sleep affects our emotions, and our emotions affect our sleep.[6] When our emotions are heightened during the day, getting adequate sleep can be harder at

night. The relationship is also a causal one. We know that greater improvements in sleep cause greater improvements in mental health and vice versa.[7]

Poor sleep on a routine basis is associated with mental health difficulties including depression, anxiety, ADHD, bipolar disorder, and others. This may be, in part, because sleep deprivation makes us more emotional and sensitive to stressful events.[8] Positive thoughts and memories are consolidated (or committed to long-term memory so that they can be recalled in the future) during REM sleep, so the impact of reduced time spent in REM can have profound emotional effects.

There's no question that fears, worries, and anxiety can mess up your sleep. We've all experienced the hamster wheel of anxious thoughts that keep sleep far out of our reach. Anxiety is a response that causes our body to activate—think fight-or-flight—so it operates in direct opposition to sleep. Anxiety motivates us for action to confront a perceived threat in our environment. As previously mentioned, it wouldn't make much sense at all to sleep in the face of a threat. Anxiety about not sleeping is really a double whammy. Anxiety increases levels of arousal, which leads to difficulty sleeping, which then results in more anxiety and worry about the loss of sleep!

The relationship between sleep and depression is quite strong.[9] A well-known symptom of depression is sleep disturbance. Sleep disturbances can take the form of sleep loss (i.e., insomnia) or too much sleep (i.e., hypersomnia). Yet research is increasingly suggesting that inadequate sleep can cause or worsen depression. Fortunately, improving sleep can also improve depression.

Adults who regularly get insufficient sleep are more likely to suffer from chronic conditions including obesity, high blood pressure, heart disease, stroke, and diabetes and are at higher risk for physical injuries. In fact, insufficient sleep has been linked to seven of the fifteen leading causes of death in the United States, including cardiovascular disease, malignant neoplasm, cerebrovascular disease, accidents, diabetes, septicaemia, and hypertension.[10]

It may come as no surprise to learn that inadequate sleep is associated with higher mortality. In comparison to adults who sleep between seven and nine hours per night, those sleeping only six to seven hours have a 7 percent higher mortality risk while those sleeping fewer than six hours have a 13 percent higher mortality risk.[11] Furthermore, adults seem to be rather inept at judging their own sleepiness. Despite knowing that they've slept fewer than the recommended number of hours of sleep, adults appear to be bad at judging when they feel tired, even when they are showing cognitive deficits including difficulty remembering, speaking, understanding, and concentrating![12] This leads us to an important tip—when it comes to sleep, trust the clock and your bedtime routine over your own judgment of wakefulness. Consider too that this less-than-perfect judgment may result in (1) inadvertently modeling for your child that sleep is not so important, and (2) having difficulty detecting when your child is tired and would benefit from more sleep.

The deficits in cognitive functioning due to sleep loss have implications for workplace productivity too. Each year, the United States loses an estimated 1.23 million working days (or 9.8 million working hours) due to insufficient sleep.[13] Estimates of the economic costs of sleep deprivation run up to $433 billion per year. If those who are sleeping fewer than six hours per night were to increase their sleep to between six and seven hours per night, the U.S. economy would increase by $226.4 billion. Now that would be a big impact!

So your sleep matters. A lot. Sleep deprivation is associated with adverse mental and physical health conditions and a higher mortality risk, along with large economic losses. Solving the problem of insufficient sleep has the potential to benefit not only one's quality of life but also the greater good of society.

Solving the Sleep Problem

Did you get enough sleep last night? Was it good quality sleep? There's a good chance that the answer to both questions is no. Seven hours of uninterrupted sleep—that's the bare minimum required for optimal functioning. So what can you do to improve your sleep quality and quantity? Read on for some relatively easy adjustments, and a few not-so-easy but doable ones, that can really add up. Recall that even a few minutes of extra sleep has been shown to improve daytime functioning.

Do More of This

1. *Keep a strict sleep schedule.* To stay in sync with your 24-hour circadian rhythm, try to go to bed and wake up at the same time each day—even on weekends. If you aren't a morning lark, get exposure to direct sunlight in the morning to help stop the production of melatonin. Sunlight is a powerful cue to help wake up and shake off that groggy feeling.[14] Eating breakfast can help to signal to your body that it's up and at 'em time too.

2. *Limit use of your bed to sleep (and sex).* Because of the power of sleep associations, things that you do in your bed (e.g., eating, work, watching TV) will become associated with your bed and not with sleep. We want sleep and your bed to be powerful partners! You can use sleep associations to your advantage too. For example, if you routinely use an aroma-therapy diffuser to scent your bedroom with lavender essential oils at night, the smell of lavender will become associated with sleep. As you settle in each night with lavender wafting through the air, your brain and body will be conditioned to respond with sleep.

3. *Prepare your sleep environment for optimal sleep.* Keep the room dark and cool with a room temperature around 60–68 degrees Fahrenheit. Black out shades and sleep

masks are helpful for reducing exposure to light. If you and your partner disagree about what makes the bedroom comfortable, see if you can reach a compromise position. For example, if you would like to sleep with an electric blanket but your partner wouldn't, find one with dual controls. Keep the bedroom quiet and turn your clock around so you won't be able to watch it if you wake up during the night. Clock watching can lead to increased anxiety and stress about not being able to sleep. Ensure your phone and other electronic devices are out of reach.

4. *Get out of bed if you can't sleep.* Do this even if the sleeplessness occurs in the middle of the night, after you've been asleep for some time. Generally, if you've been lying in bed for more than fifteen minutes, it's time to get up, out of bed, and do something quiet, relaxing, and otherwise non-stimulating. Meditation, mindful deep breathing, progressive muscle relaxation, reading a book, listening to quiet music or an audiobook are a few good options. You'll want to choose a nonfiction book over a gripping whodunit! Go back to bed only when you are feeling sleepy again. This helps to build that important association between your bed and sleep and to eliminate the unwanted association between your bed and wakefulness. For more on this, see the upcoming section titled "Middle-of-the-Night Awakenings."

5. *Devote time during the day to manage your stressors.* To avoid the onslaught of worried thoughts as you lie down to go to sleep, give yourself some time during the day to address these concerns. Sometimes, just putting thoughts to paper can put them to bed (no pun intended!). Once they are in print, you may feel the benefit of a reduced mental load or "worry work" (the invisible mental effort it takes to manage such thoughts). Other times, problem-solving around the issue is needed to leave you feeling more in control of the

situation. Recording these thoughts in a journal or note-book can help you to organize them, gain some objectivity from them, and brainstorm potential solutions. Once your thoughts are written out, worries can seem less plausible and more manageable. The truth is that most of our anxious thoughts are not perfectly rational and, as research suggests, 85 percent of our worries result in a neutral or positive outcome.[15] We like those odds!

You might also consider devoting a set time to think about your worries and stressful thoughts. Indulge them only during that time frame, for example, 3:00–3:30 p.m. Keep the "worry time" earlier in the day, not in the evening. When your half hour of "worry time" is up, move your thoughts along. You're done with worries. If you find yourself unable to keep your anxious or stressful thoughts from interfering with your day, consider psychological therapy. Cognitive-behavioral therapy has been demonstrated to be very effective for anxiety, insomnia, and numerous other problems. Most health insurance plans cover treatment costs, at least in part, and virtual therapy sessions are widely available. You don't even need to leave your home. Now, that's convenient!

6. *Enjoy a wind-down routine at the end of the day.* Bedtime routines aren't just for kids! Though it may be difficult, make the time to engage in some relaxing activities that help you to wind down for the night. Taking a hot bath or shower, reading, eating a light snack, or engaging in a relaxing hobby are great elements to add to your routine. Your bedroom, and most importantly, your bed, should be reserved for sleeping so you may wish to find a quiet place for your evening routine elsewhere in your home.

7. *Get daily exercise.* Even small amounts of exercise have been shown to improve sleep. The exercise doesn't even have to be strenuous. Moderate exercise, such as walking, roller skating,

and tai chi, was found to be more effective at improving sleep quality than vigorous exercise.[16] It's a win-win—you'll sleep better and improve your physical health. Exercise early in the day because physical activity close to bedtime can disrupt your sleep. Leave a window of about four hours between your exercise and your bedtime.

8. *Keep track of your sleep with a sleep diary.* If you are someone who struggles with getting enough sleep, learn more about the quality and quantity of your sleep as well as what influences it—for better or worse—using a sleep diary. Sleep diaries allow you to track information such as when you fell asleep, how long it took, how many times you woke up during the night, as well as how rested you felt, whether you napped during the day, took medication, or used substances. The National Heart, Lung, and Blood Institute has developed a sleep diary that is in the public domain and free to access at https://www.nhlbi.nih.gov/resources/sleep-diary. Gathering these details across several weeks (or longer) can help you to identify your sleep patterns and uncover the reasons behind your sleep difficulties.

If logging your sleep seems too time-consuming, consider use of a sleep tracking device. Sleep trackers can be wearable (e.g., headband, wristband, ring), devices that lay on or under your mattress, or even smart phone apps that gather a variety of sleep data including time awake, time in each of the sleep stages, snoring, sleep talking, and more. Sleep trackers work by using built-in accelerometers or sonar that track your breathing rate, heart rate, or body movements to assess your sleep data. The data is then uploaded, analyzed, and reported back to you, often with individualized sleep recommendations based on your personal data. The devices are generally reliable and becoming more sophisticated and specialized over time.

And Less of This

1. *Use of caffeine, nicotine, exercise, and screens before bed.* To provide a safe buffer zone, limit or avoid caffeine use after 1 p.m. Be sure to check for caffeine in the products that you consume. You may be surprised by the amount of caffeine they contain. Because caffeine stays in your body for a long time, significant amounts of caffeine may still be exerting a stimulating effect many hours after consumption, right as you are trying to sleep. Similarly, cutting down or stopping nicotine use is also helpful to get a better night's rest. While nicotine might seem to help you relax, it is a stimulant that is counterproductive when you are trying to sleep. Exercise earlier in the day, since exercise at night can have an arousing effect. Similarly, recall that the blue light from screens can make your brain think it's daytime, shutting down many of the body's natural sleep preparations.

2. *Alcohol before bed.* Many people believe that alcohol use is a good option for aiding in sleep; however, this is not the case. Alcohol before bed is problematic for several reasons. It is true that you may fall asleep much faster when under its influence. During the first half of the night, alcohol will have a calming effect, ushering you into a dreamless sleep. However, during the second half of the night, as the alcohol level in your body begins to decrease, you'll likely have a fragmented night of sleep—rife with stressful dreams and frequent awakenings. Since alcohol is a diuretic, you'll experience an increased need to urinate, and due to its muscle-relaxing properties affecting your upper airways, you'll snore more. It's especially important to avoid mixing alcohol, a central nervous system depressant, with other sedating medications such as prescription sleep medications, pain-relieving sleep aids (e.g., Advil PM), melatonin, or antihistamines (e.g., Benadryl). If you wish to drink alcohol in the evenings, try to do so no later than four or more hours before bedtime.

3. *Afternoon napping, especially if you are someone who has difficulty sleeping at night.* Don't nap after 2 p.m. and not longer
than twenty or twenty-five minutes. Any longer and you'll
risk entering the deeper stages of sleep. Waking from deep
sleep can leave you with a "sleep hangover" in which you'll
feel more tired than before you took the nap! In addition, an
afternoon nap can reduce your need to sleep in the evening
hours, making it harder to fall asleep. The closer the nap is
to bedtime, the more likely it is that you've used up some
of your "sleep drive," your body's natural push to fall asleep
at night. If you skip the nap altogether, your body's natural
drive to fall asleep at bedtime will be high, and you'll be
sufficiently sleepy when you crawl into bed at night.

What about Sleep Aids?

Sleep aids are over-the-counter (OTC) or prescription medications that can be effective for achieving more sleep. In general,
their use should be limited to a night here or there. A reliance on
sleep aids is not likely to be a good long-term solution for poor
sleep. Most of the OTC sleep aids rely on the sedating effects of
antihistamines. Though antihistamines can induce sleepiness, they
can also result in morning grogginess and, over time, it is possible
to develop tolerance, necessitating more and more of the antihis-
tamine to produce the same effect.

Recall, melatonin supplements are often used to help with sleep
due to their influence on the sleep-wake cycle. They can help one to
fall asleep faster but don't tend to help one stay asleep. Melatonin
supplements have also been associated with headaches or nausea in
some individuals, and they typically have only a mild effect on sleep.
Because melatonin supplementation can lengthen the time spent in
REM sleep (when we dream), it can result in a greater number of
vivid dreams or nightmares. As noted earlier in this book, melatonin
supplements are not regulated by the FDA, leading to uncertainty
about how much and exactly what you are getting in each dose.

Cannabis, also known as marijuana, and cannabidiol (CBD), a compound derived from the cannabis plant, have been widely touted as remedies for a wide variety of conditions including insomnia. While some research has been suggestive of the benefits of cannabinoids in the treatment of sleep difficulties, the research is preliminary. It may be that any improvements in sleep are a byproduct of the cannabinoids' effects on anxiety or pain, thus enabling one to sleep better.[17] Authors of a recent study examining the utility of cannabinoids in the treatment of sleep disorders concluded that there is insufficient evidence to suggest routine use of cannabinoids to treat sleep problems, noting the lack of quality, large-scale, and unbiased published research studies.[18] So the jury's still out on this one.

If you have tried all the strategies described herein and sleep continues to elude you, it might be time to consult with your doctor. Prescription sleep medications (often referred to as sleeping pills) are available and effective, especially for short-term use. Sleeping pill use is associated with side effects (e.g., daytime drowsiness, dizziness, dry mouth, headaches, digestive problems) and can lead to tolerance so that you need more of the drug to have the same effect. Talk with your doctor to find the best intervention to help you rest easy.

MIDDLE-OF-THE-NIGHT AWAKENINGS

It's normal to wake up sometimes in the middle of the night, and it should be easy to go back to sleep. In the morning, you might not even remember that you woke during the night.

Here are a few strategies you can use to get back to sleep. Try them all and see which work best for you.

- As noted earlier, get out of bed if you wake in the middle of the night and find yourself unable to return to sleep after fifteen minutes. While out of bed, choose an activity that is low key, boring, or relaxing. Don't pay bills or catch up on work, which can be stressful. Avoid screens, so playing on your phone and watching TV are not good options. Folding laundry, reading, praying, listening to calming music, visualizing a favorite location, or mentally reviewing a pleasant time in your life are a few good activities to try when you find yourself unable to sleep. Just remember to leave your bed when you engage in them. You want to do all you can to preserve the association between sleep and your bed by doing nothing but sleeping in your bed.

- Light stretches are a great way to soothe and relax your body. Stretching reduces muscle tension and increases serotonin, a good mood hormone. Relaxation exercises can be helpful too. Try a full body scan, noticing where your body feels tense. Moving from head to toes, draw your attention to each muscle group (face, neck, shoulders, back, abdomen, legs, feet) and intentionally relax the muscles. It is sometimes helpful to flex or tense a muscle group and then release the tension to ensure that the muscles are loose and relaxed. These are the same progressive muscle relaxation (PMR) exercises that you did with your child in Week 3. They work for adults too!

- Try some meditation. Meditation has been linked to more and higher-quality sleep. In a study of individuals with chronic insomnia, those who practiced eight weeks of meditation slept nearly forty-five minutes more than those who did not.[19] If you've never practiced meditation before, there are a number of apps to help you get started. Calm and Headspace are two popular apps for guided meditation. A word to the wise, practicing meditation takes effort and concentration, so don't expect relaxation or immediate proficiency at staying focused.

- Do some focused breathing exercises. Breathe in to the count of one; breathe out to the count of two. Count to twenty and repeat as needed. We predict you'll have a hard time making it past the first round of twenty! If you find that your mind is wandering away from the count, gently bring the focus back to your breath and restart. Placing the focus on your breathing does a great job of preventing any worrisome or stressful thoughts from creeping in. Research has shown that breathing exercises can lower blood pressure, slow heart rate, and reduce stress.

When Nothing Seems to Work . . .

If you've tried these strategies and are still having trouble getting enough hours of quality sleep, consult with a sleep expert. Consider an evaluation for an underlying condition (e.g., a sleep disorder). Whether you are diagnosed with another condition or not, you might benefit from cognitive-behavioral therapy for insomnia (CBTi). CBTi is a short-term, research-supported intervention that is effective for both short-term and chronic insomnia that works by targeting the thoughts, feelings, and behaviors that are contributing to insufficient sleep. In-person and online CBTi options are available. Research finds that even a single session of CBTi can be beneficial.[20] You can download the free app, CBT-i Coach, offered by the U.S. Department of Veterans Affairs, to provide psychological guidance on combating insomnia. Use of the app is intended to accompany therapy with a health professional.

Oversleeping: Too Much of a Good Thing

Though less of a problem for many, research has demonstrated that consistently getting too much sleep is associated with a variety of negative health effects. Oversleeping (more than nine hours a night) has been linked to an increased risk of disease (e.g., coronary heart disease, obesity, diabetes). It's a Goldilocks situation—neither too little nor too much sleep. Seven to nine hours per night is just right. Oversleeping can also indicate an underlying problem, so consult with your doctor if you routinely sleep more than nine hours a night.

Benefits of Increased Sleep

When you sleep well, a myriad of benefits will reveal themselves. You'll enjoy more energy, a better mood, enhanced concentration and creativity, less sickness, and less stress. An additional benefit is the positive impact your quality sleep will have on your child's sleep. Your child's sleep will improve. It's not magic, it's modeling! When you make a commitment to ensuring sufficient and high-quality sleep for yourself, you are modeling this value to your child. Your child will learn to appreciate the importance of sleep. When everyone in the home sees the benefits of some serious shut-eye, moods and relationships are improved and bedtimes are easier. We don't mean to say that adequate sleep will solve all the world's problems, but we bet it will make a serious dent.

So now that you and your child are getting adequate sleep and bedtimes are short, sweet, and battle-free, what amazing things will you do with the extra time on your hands?

 Now Apply It!

1. Complete a sleep diary. Download the National Heart, Lung, and Blood Institute's sleep diary at https:// www.nhlbi.nih.gov/resources/sleep-diary or find an alternative sleep diary online. Track your sleep data for several weeks to uncover patterns, sleep disruptors, and factors that help you to achieve quality sleep.

2. Engage in practices that enhance your sleep. Spend some time creating an inviting sleep environment, and develop routines using information that you uncover using your sleep diary.

Bonus Week Summary

- Build a daily schedule that includes a consistent wake time and bedtime, moderate exercise, and an end-of-the-day wind-down period, and results in about seven to nine hours of sleep per night.

- Maximize the association between sleep and your bed. Limit use of the bed to sleep and sexual activity only. Prepare your sleep environment to limit factors that interfere with sleep (e.g., light, noise) and increase the factors that promote sleep (e.g., cool temperature in bedroom). If you find yourself unable to sleep, get out of bed and engage in a quiet, relaxing, and nontaxing activity such as reading, praying, or listening to soft music.

- Manage your stressors during the day so that you reduce your chances of dwelling on them as you lay in bed at night. Use of a worry journal, designated "worry time," or psychotherapy are good options for alleviating stress and anxiety.

- Learn more about your sleep using a sleep diary. Track information such as when you fell asleep, how long it took, how many times you woke up during the night, as well as how rested you felt, whether you napped during the day, took medication, or used substances. Learn what factors optimize your sleep and which ones detract from it.

- Limit your use of substances and activities that have an arousing effect on the body. These include caffeine, nicotine, exercise late in the day, and electronic devices. Be wary of afternoon naps as well because they can lessen your body's desire for sleep in the evening.

- Sleep aids include over-the-counter or prescription medications or products that are used to improve the amount and quality of sleep. In general, their use should be limited to the short-term. If you believe that you need help in increasing the amount or quality of your sleep, consult with your doctor about the sleep aids that are best for you.

- If you wake up in the middle of the night, be sure to get out of bed to retain a strong association between your bed and sleep. Engage in a relaxing or even boring task. Light stretching, meditation, and breathing exercises can also be helpful in getting you back to sleep.

- If all your attempts to improve your sleep on your own have not gotten you the sleep you deserve, consider cognitive-behavioral therapy for insomnia (CBTi). CBTi is a short-term, research-based intervention that is effective for both short-term and chronic insomnia and works by targeting the thoughts, feelings, and behaviors that are contributing to insufficient sleep.

- Oversleeping (more than nine hours a night) has been linked to a variety of negative health effects. Aim for seven to nine hours of sleep per night.

Sleep Resources for Parents

American Academy of Child and Adolescent Psychiatry. "Sleep Problems." https://www.aacap.org/AACAP/Families_and_Youth /Facts_for_Families/FFF-Guide/Childrens-Sleep-Problems-034 .aspx.

American Academy of Family Physicians. "What You Need to Know about Sleep for Your Child." https://www.aafp.org/pubs/ afp/issues/2022/0200/p168-s1.html.

American Academy of Pediatrics. "Safe Sleep." https://www.aap .org/en/patient-care/safe-sleep/.

American Academy of Pediatrics—Healthy Children Website. https://www.healthychildren.org/.

American Academy of Sleep Medicine (Directory of Sleep Centers). https://sleepeducation.org/sleep-center/.

American Psychological Association. "Helping Children Get a Good Night's Sleep." https://www.apa.org/monitor/2020/07/ce -corner-sleep.

Centers for Disease Control and Prevention. "Do Your Children Get Enough Sleep?" and "Basics about Sleep." https://www.cdc

.gov/chronicdisease/resources/infographic/children-sleep.htm; https://www.cdc.gov/sleep/about_sleep/index.html.

Mental Health Foundation. "Sleep Guide for Parents and Care-givers." https://www.mentalhealth.org.uk/sites/default/files/2022 -06/Sleep-Guide-for-Parents-and-Caregivers.pdf.

National Sleep Foundation. https://www.thensf.org/.

Sleep Foundation. https://www.sleepfoundation.org/.

Sleep Junkies. https://sleepjunkies.com/.

Society of Behavioral Sleep Medicine (Directory of CBTi pro-viders). https://www.behavioralsleep.org/index.php/united-states -sbsm-members.

Notes

Introduction

1. V. Niark Durand and Jodi A. Mindell, "Behavioral Treatment of Multiple Childhood Sleep Disorders: Effects on Child and Family," *Behavior Modification* 14, no. 1 (1990): 37–49.

2. Andre Kahn et al., "Sleep Problems in Healthy Preadolescents," *Pediatrics* 84, no. 3 (1989): 542–46; Sarah Blunden et al., "Behavior and Neurocognitive Performance in Children Aged 5–10 Years Who Snore Compared to Controls," *Journal of Clinical and Experimental Neuropsychology* 22, no. 5 (2000): 554–68; Judith A. Owens, Anthony Spirito, Melissa McGuinn, and Chantelle Nobile, "Sleep Habits and Sleep Disturbance in Elementary School-Aged Children," *Journal of Developmental and Behavioral Pediatrics* 21, no. 1 (2000): 27–36; Robert E. Roberts, Catherine R. Roberts, and Irene G. Chen, "Functioning of Adolescents with Symptoms of Disturbed Sleep," *Journal of Youth and Adolescence* 30, no. 1 (2001): 1–18.

Week 1

1. Sarah Morsbach Honaker and Taylor Saunders, "The Sleep Checkup: Sleep Screening, Guidance, and Management in Pediatric Primary Care," *Clinical Practice in Pediatric Psychology* 6, no. 3 (2018): 201.

2. Adam T. Newton, Sarah M. Honaker, and Graham J. Reid, "Risk and Protective Factors and Processes for Behavioral Sleep Problems Among Preschool and Early School-Aged Children: A Systematic Review," *Sleep Medicine Reviews* 52 (2020): 101303.

3. Marc Weissbluth, *Healthy Sleep Habits, Happy Child: A Step-by-Step Program for a Good Night's Sleep* (New York: Ballantine Books, 2021).

4. Lisa J. Meltzer, Courtney Johnson, Jonathan Crosette, Mark Ramos, and Jodi A. Mindell, "Prevalence of Diagnosed Sleep Disorders in Pediatric Primary Care Practices," *Pediatrics* 125, no. 6 (2010): e1410–e1418.

5. Prajakta Deshpande, Betzy Salcedo, and Cynthia Haq, "Common Sleep Disorders in Children," *American Family Physician* 105, no. 2 (2022): 168–76.

6. John A. Fleetham and Jonathan A. E. Fleming, "Parasomnias," *Canadian Medical Association Journal* 186, no. 8 (2014): E273–E280; Suresh Kotagal, "Parasomnias in Childhood," *Sleep Medicine Reviews* 13, no. 2 (2009): 157–68.

7. Kevin A. Carter, Nathanael E. Hathaway, and Christine F. Lettieri, "Common Sleep Disorders in Children," *American Family Physician* 89, no. 5 (2014): 368–77.

8. G. Klackenberg, "Incidence of Parasomnias in Children in a General Population," in *Sleep and Its Disorders in Children*, ed. C. Guilleminault (Newark, DE: Raven Press, 1987): 99–113.

9. Patrina H. Y. Caldwell, Elisabeth Hodson, Jonathan C. Craig, and Denise Edgar, "4. Bedwetting and Toileting Problems in Children," *Medical Journal of Australia* 182, no. 4 (2005): 190–95.

10. Cathryn M. A. Glazener, Jonathan H. C. Evans, and Rachel E. Peto, "Alarm Interventions for Nocturnal Enuresis in Children," *Cochrane Database of Systematic Reviews* 2 (2005).

11. Glazener et al., "Alarm Interventions for Nocturnal Enuresis in Children."

12. Deshpande et al., "Common Sleep Disorders in Children," 168.

13. Carter et al., "Common Sleep Disorders in Children," 368.

14. Robert L. Sack et al., "Circadian Rhythm Sleep Disorders: Part II, Advanced Sleep Phase Disorder, Delayed Sleep Phase Disorder, Free-Running Disorder, and Irregular Sleep-Wake Rhythm," *Sleep* 30, no. 11 (2007): 1484–501.

15. Nathaniel F. Watson et al., "Delaying Middle School and High School Start Times Promotes Student Health and Performance: An American Academy of Sleep Medicine Position Statement," *Journal of Clinical Sleep Medicine* 13, no. 4 (2017): 623–25.

16. Eric Suni and A. Singh, "How Much Sleep Do We Really Need," *Sleep Foundation* (2021).

17. Jodi A. Mindell and Ariel A. Williamson, "Benefits of a Bedtime Routine in Young Children: Sleep, Development, and Beyond," *Sleep Medicine Reviews* 40 (2018): 93–108.

18. Lisa A. Adams and Vaughn I. Rickert, "Reducing Bedtime Tantrums: Comparison between Positive Routines and Graduated Extinction," *Pediatrics* 84, no. 5 (1989): 756–61.

19. Edward C. Harding, Nicholas P. Franks, and William Wisden, "The Temperature Dependence of Sleep," *Frontiers in Neuroscience* 13 (2019): 336.

20. Tiffany Field, Maria Hernandez-Reif, Miguel Diego, Saul Schanberg, and Cynthia Kuhn, "Cortisol Decreases and Serotonin and Dopamine Increase Following Massage Therapy," *International Journal of Neuroscience* 115, no. 10 (2005): 1397–413.

21. Nomathemba Dube, Kaviul Khan, Sarah Loehr, Yen Chu, and Paul Veugelers, "The Use of Entertainment and Communication Technologies before

Sleep Could Affect Sleep and Weight Status: A Population-Based Study among Children," *International Journal of Behavioral Nutrition and Physical Activity* 14 (2017): 1–15.

22. Steven W. Lockley, George C. Brainard, and Charles A. Czeisler, "High Sensitivity of the Human Circadian Melatonin Rhythm to Resetting by Short Wavelength Light," *Journal of Clinical Endocrinology & Metabolism* 88, no. 9 (2003): 4502–5.

23. Pieter A. Cohen, Bharathi Avula, Yan-Hong Wang, Kumar Katragunta, and Ikhlas Khan, "Quantity of Melatonin and CBD in Melatonin Gummies Sold in the US," *Journal of the American Medical Association* 329, no. 16 (2023): 1401–2.

24. Cohen et al., "Quantity of Melatonin and CBD in Melatonin Gummies," 1401.

25. Megan Witbracht, Nancy L. Keim, Shavawn Forester, Adrianne Widaman, and Kevin Laugero, "Female Breakfast Skippers Display a Disrupted Cortisol Rhythm and Elevated Blood Pressure," *Physiology & Behavior* 140 (2015): 215–21.

26. U.S. Department of Health and Human Services, *Physical Activity Guidelines for Americans*, 2nd ed. (Washington, DC: U.S. Department of Health and Human Services, 2018).

27. Gillian M. Nixon et al., "Falling Asleep: The Determinants of Sleep Latency," *Archives of Disease in Childhood* 94, no. 9 (2009): 686–89.

28. Anna M. H. Price, Melissa Wake, Obioha C. Ukoumunne, and Harriet Hiscock, "Five-Year Follow-Up of Harms and Benefits of Behavioral Infant Sleep Intervention: Randomized Trial," *Pediatrics* 130, no. 4 (2012): 643–51.

WEEK 2

1. Terrence Sanvictores and Magda D. Mendez, "Types of Parenting Styles and Effects on Children" (2021), StatPearls, PMID: 33760502.

2. Lauren B. Covington et al., "The Contributory Role of the Family Context in Early Childhood Sleep Health: A Systematic Review," *Sleep Health* 7, no. 2 (2021): 254–65.

WEEK 3

1. Ciro Conversano et al., "Mindfulness, Age and Gender as Protective Factors against Psychological Distress during COVID-19 Pandemic," *Frontiers in Psychology* 11 (2020): 1900.

2. Arlene S. Koeppen, "Relaxation Training for Children," *Elementary School Guidance & Counseling* 9, no. 1 (1974): 14–21.

Week 4

1. Ann E. Bigelow and Lela Rankin Williams, "To Have and to Hold: Effects of Physical Contact on Infants and Their Caregivers," *Infant Behavior and Development* 61 (2020): 101494.

2. Brett K. Jakubiak and Brooke C. Feeney, "Affectionate Touch to Promote Relational, Psychological, and Physical Well-Being in Adulthood: A Theoretical Model and Review of the Research," *Personality and Social Psychology Review* 21, no. 3 (2017): 228–52.

3. Reut Gruber, Jamie Cassoff, Sonia Frenette, Sabrina Wiebe, and Julie Carrier, "Impact of Sleep Extension and Restriction on Children's Emotional Lability and Impulsivity," *Pediatrics* 130, no. 5 (2012): e1155–e1161; Reut Gruber, Gail Somerville, Lana Bergmame, Laura Fontil, and Soukaina Paquin, "School-Based Sleep Education Program Improves Sleep and Academic Performance of School-Age Children," *Sleep Medicine* 21 (2016): 93–100.

Week 5

1. Gail Hornor et al., "Building a Safe and Healthy America: Eliminating Corporal Punishment via Positive Parenting," *Journal of Pediatric Health Care* 34, no. 2 (2020): 136–44.

2. Elizabeth T. Gershoff, *Report on Physical Punishment in the United States: What Research Tells Us about Its Effects on Children* (Columbus, OH: Center for Effective Discipline, 2008).

Bonus Week

1. David Richter, Michael D. Krämer, Nicole K. Y. Tang, Hawley E. Montgomery-Downs, and Sakari Lemola, "Long-Term Effects of Pregnancy and Childbirth on Sleep Satisfaction and Duration of First-Time and Experienced Mothers and Fathers," *Sleep* 42, no. 4 (2019): zsz015.

2. Yong Liu, Anne G. Wheaton, Daniel P. Chapman, Timothy J. Cunningham, Hua Lu, and Janet B. Croft, "Prevalence of Healthy Sleep Duration among Adults—United States, 2014," *Morbidity and Mortality Weekly Report* 65, no. 6 (2016): 137–41.

3. Sarah Berger, "What Time Elon Musk, Barack Obama and 4 Other Successful People Go to Bed," CNBC, June 22, 2018, https://www.cnbc.com/2018/06/22/what-time-successful-people-to-go-bed.html.

4. Berger, "What Time Elon Musk, Barack Obama . . . Go to Bed."

5. "Donald Trump Quotes," accessed October 6, 2023, http://www.quoteswise.com/donald-trump-quotes-6.html.

6. Seithikurippu R. Pandi-Perumal et al., "Clarifying the Role of Sleep in Depression: A Narrative Review," *Psychiatry Research* 291 (2020): 113239.

7. Alexander J. Scott, Thomas L. Webb, Marrissa Martyn-St James, Georgina Rowse, and Scott Weich, "Improving Sleep Quality Leads to Better Mental

Health: A Meta-Analysis of Randomised Controlled Trials," *Sleep Medicine Reviews* 60 (2021): 101556; Daniel J. Schwartz, William C. Kohler, and Gillian Karatinos, "Symptoms of Depression in Individuals with Obstructive Sleep Apnea May Be Amenable to Treatment with Continuous Positive Airway Pressure," *Chest* 128, no. 3 (2005): 1304–9.

8. Marie Vandekerckhove and Yu-lin Wang, "Emotion, Emotion Regulation and Sleep: An Intimate Relationship," *AIMS Neuroscience* 5, no. 1 (2018): 1.

9. David Nutt, Sue Wilson, and Louise Paterson, "Sleep Disorders as Core Symptoms of Depression," *Dialogues in Clinical Neuroscience* (2022).

10. Kenneth D. Kochanek, *Mortality in the United States, 2013*, no. 178, U.S. Department of Health and Human Services, Centers for Disease Control and Prevention, National Center for Health Statistics, 2014.

11. Marco Hafner, Martin Stepanek, Jirka Taylor, Wendy M. Troxel, and Christian van Stolk, "Why Sleep Matters—The Economic Costs of Insufficient Sleep: A Cross-Country Comparative Analysis," *RAND Health Quarterly* 6, no. 4 (2017).

12. Hans P. A. Van Dongen, Greg Maislin, Janet M. Mullington, and David F. Dinges, "The Cumulative Cost of Additional Wakefulness: Dose-Response Effects on Neurobehavioral Functions and Sleep Physiology from Chronic Sleep Restriction and Total Sleep Deprivation," *Sleep* 26, no. 2 (2003): 117–26.

13. Hafner et al., "Why Sleep Matters."

14. Mariana G. Figueiro et al., "The Impact of Daytime Light Exposures on Sleep and Mood in Office Workers," *Sleep Health* 3, no. 3 (2017): 204–15.

15. T. D. Borkovec, Holly Hazlett-Stevens, and M. L. Diaz. "The Role of Positive Beliefs about Worry in Generalized Anxiety Disorder and Its Treatment," *Clinical Psychology & Psychotherapy: An International Journal of Theory & Practice* 6, no. 2 (1999): 126–38.

16. Feifei Wang and Szilvia Boros, "The Effect of Physical Activity on Sleep Quality: A Systematic Review," *European Journal of Physiotherapy* 23, no. 1 (2021): 11–18.

17. Lucile Rapin, Rihab Gamaoun, Cynthia El Hage, Maria Fernanda Arboleda, and Erin Prosk, "Cannabidiol Use and Effectiveness: Real-World Evidence from a Canadian Medical Cannabis Clinic," *Journal of Cannabis Research* 3, no. 1 (2021): 1–10.

18. Anastasia S. Suraev et al., "Cannabinoid Therapies in the Management of Sleep Disorders: A Systematic Review of Preclinical and Clinical Studies," *Sleep Medicine Reviews* 53 (2020): 101339.

19. Jason C. Ong, Rachel Manber, Zindel Segal, Yinglin Xia, Shauna Shapiro, and James K. Wyatt, "A Randomized Controlled Trial of Mindfulness Meditation for Chronic Insomnia," *Sleep* 37, no. 9 (2014): 1553–63.

20. Jason G. Ellis, Toby Cushing, and Anne Germain, "Treating Acute Insomnia: A Randomized Controlled Trial of a 'Single-Shot' of Cognitive Behavioral Therapy for Insomnia," *Sleep* 38, no. 6 (2015): 971–78.

Bibliography

Adams, Lisa A., and Vaughn I. Rickert. "Reducing Bedtime Tantrums: Comparison Between Positive Routines and Graduated Extinction." *Pediatrics* 84, no. 5 (1989): 756–61.

Berger, Sarah. "What Time Elon Musk, Barack Obama and 4 Other Successful People Go to Bed." CNBC, June 22, 2018. https://www.cnbc.com/2018/06/22/what-time-successful-people-to-go-bed.html.

Bigelow, Ann E., and Lela Rankin Williams. "To Have and to Hold: Effects of Physical Contact on Infants and Their Caregivers." *Infant Behavior and Development* 61 (2020): 101494.

Blunden, Sarah, Kurt Lushington, Declan Kennedy, James Martin, and Drew Dawson. "Behavior and Neurocognitive Performance in Children Aged 5–10 Years Who Snore Compared to Controls." *Journal of Clinical and Experimental Neuropsychology* 22, no. 5 (2000): 554–68.

Borkovec, T. D., Holly Hazlett-Stevens, and M. L. Diaz. "The Role of Positive Beliefs about Worry in Generalized Anxiety Disorder and Its Treatment." *Clinical Psychology & Psychotherapy: An International Journal of Theory & Practice* 6, no. 2 (1999): 126–38.

Caldwell, Patrina H. Y., Elisabeth Hodson, Jonathan C. Craig, and Denise Edgar. "4. Bedwetting and Toileting Problems in Children." *Medical Journal of Australia* 182, no. 4 (2005): 190–95.

Carter, Kevin A., Nathanael E. Hathaway, and Christine F. Lettieri. "Common Sleep Disorders in Children." *American Family Physician* 89, no. 5 (2014): 368–77.

Cohen, Pieter A., Bharathi Avula, Yan-Hong Wang, Kumar Katragunta, and Ikhlas Khan. "Quantity of Melatonin and CBD in Melatonin Gummies Sold in the US." *Journal of the American Medical Association* 329, no. 16 (2023): 1401–2.

Conversano, Ciro, Mariagrazia Di Giuseppe, Mario Miccoli, Rebecca Ciacchini, Angelo Gemignani, and Graziella Orrù. "Mindfulness, Age and Gender as Protective Factors against Psychological Distress during COVID-19 Pandemic." *Frontiers in Psychology* 11 (2020): 1900.

Covington, Lauren B., Freda Patterson, Lauren E. Hale, Douglas M. Teti, Angeni Cordova, Shannon Mayberry, and Emily J. Hauenstein. "The Contributory Role of the Family Context in Early Childhood Sleep Health: A Systematic Review." *Sleep Health* 7, no. 2 (2021): 254–65.

Deshpande, Prajakta, Betzy Salcedo, and Cynthia Haq. "Common Sleep Disorders in Children." *American Family Physician* 105, no. 2 (2022): 168–76.

Dube, Nomathemba, Kaviul Khan, Sarah Loehr, Yen Chu, and Paul Veugelers. "The Use of Entertainment and Communication Technologies before Sleep Could Affect Sleep and Weight Status: A Population-Based Study among Children." *International Journal of Behavioral Nutrition and Physical Activity* 14 (2017): 1–15.

Durand, V. Niark, and Jodi A. Mindell. "Behavioral Treatment of Multiple Childhood Sleep Disorders: Effects on Child and Family." *Behavior Modification* 14, no. 1 (1990): 37–49.

Ellis, Jason G., Toby Cushing, and Anne Germain. "Treating Acute Insomnia: A Randomized Controlled Trial of a 'Single-Shot' of Cognitive Behavioral Therapy for Insomnia." *Sleep* 38, no. 6 (2015): 971–78.

Field, Tiffany, Maria Hernandez-Reif, Miguel Diego, Saul Schanberg, and Cynthia Kuhn. "Cortisol Decreases and Serotonin and Dopamine Increase following Massage Therapy." *International Journal of Neuroscience* 115, no. 10 (2005): 1397–413.

Figueiro, Mariana G., Bryan Steverson, Judith Heerwagen, Kevin Kampschroer, Claudia M. Hunter, Kassandra Gonzales, Barbara Plitnick, and Mark S. Rea. "The Impact of Daytime Light Exposures on Sleep and Mood in Office Workers." *Sleep Health* 3, no. 3 (2017): 204–15.

Fleetham, John A., and Jonathan A. E. Fleming. "Parasomnias." *Canadian Medical Association Journal* 186, no. 8 (2014): E273–E280.

Gershoff, Elizabeth T. *Report on Physical Punishment in the United States: What Research Tells Us about Its Effects on Children.* Columbus, OH: Center for Effective Discipline, 2008.

Glazener, Cathryn M. A., Jonathan H. C. Evans, and Rachel E. Peto. "Alarm Interventions for Nocturnal Enuresis in Children." *Cochrane Database of Systematic Reviews* 2 (2005).

Gruber, Reut, Jamie Cassoff, Sonia Frenette, Sabrina Wiebe, and Julie Carrier. "Impact of Sleep Extension and Restriction on Children's Emotional Lability and Impulsivity." *Pediatrics* 130, no. 5 (2012): e1155–e1161.

Gruber, Reut, Gail Somerville, Lana Bergmame, Laura Fontil, and Soukaina Paquin. "School-Based Sleep Education Program Improves Sleep and Academic Performance of School-Age Children." *Sleep Medicine* 21 (2016): 93–100.

Hafner, Marco, Martin Stepanek, Jirka Taylor, Wendy M. Troxel, and Christian van Stolk. "Why Sleep Matters—The Economic Costs of Insufficient

Sleep: A Cross-Country Comparative Analysis." *RAND Health Quarterly* 6, no. 4 (2017).

Harding, Edward C., Nicholas P. Franks, and William Wisden. "The Temperature Dependence of Sleep." *Frontiers in Neuroscience* 13 (2019): 336.

Honaker, Sarah Morsbach, and Taylor Saunders. "The Sleep Checkup: Sleep Screening, Guidance, and Management in Pediatric Primary Care." *Clinical Practice in Pediatric Psychology* 6, no. 3 (2018): 201.

Hornor, Gail, Saribel Garcia Quinones, Danielle Boudreaux, Deborah Bretl, Evelyn Chapman, Ellen M. Chiocca, Carrie Donnell et al. "Building a Safe and Healthy America: Eliminating Corporal Punishment via Positive Parenting." *Journal of Pediatric Health Care* 34, no. 2 (2020): 136–44.

Jakubiak, Brett K., and Brooke C. Feeney. "Affectionate Touch to Promote Relational, Psychological, and Physical Well-Being in Adulthood: A Theoretical Model and Review of the Research." *Personality and Social Psychology Review* 21, no. 3 (2017): 228–52.

Kahn, Andre, Carine Van de Merckt, Elisabeth Rebuffat, Marie Jose Mozin, Martine Sottiaux, Denise Blum, and Philippe Hennart. "Sleep Problems in Healthy Preadolescents." *Pediatrics* 84, no. 3 (1989): 542–46.

Klackenberg, G. "Incidence of Parasomnias in Children in a General Population." In *Sleep and Its Disorders in Children*, edited by C. Guilleminault, 99–113. Newark, DE: Raven Press, 1987.

Kochanek, Kenneth D. *Mortality in the United States, 2013.* No. 178. U.S. Department of Health and Human Services, Centers for Disease Control and Prevention, National Center for Health Statistics, 2014.

Koeppen, Arlene S. "Relaxation Training for Children." *Elementary School Guidance & Counseling* 9, no. 1 (1974): 14–21.

Kotagal, Suresh. "Parasomnias in Childhood." *Sleep Medicine Reviews* 13, no. 2 (2009): 157–68.

Liu, Yong, Anne G. Wheaton, Daniel P. Chapman, Timothy J. Cunningham, Hua Lu, and Janet B. Croft. "Prevalence of Healthy Sleep Duration among Adults—United States, 2014." *Morbidity and Mortality Weekly Report* 65, no. 6 (2016): 137–41.

Lockley, Steven W., George C. Brainard, and Charles A. Czeisler. "High Sensitivity of the Human Circadian Melatonin Rhythm to Resetting by Short Wavelength Light." *Journal of Clinical Endocrinology & Metabolism* 88, no. 9 (2003): 4502–5.

Meltzer, Lisa J., Courtney Johnson, Jonathan Crosette, Mark Ramos, and Jodi A. Mindell. "Prevalence of Diagnosed Sleep Disorders in Pediatric Primary Care Practices." *Pediatrics* 125, no. 6 (2010): e1410–e1418.

Mindell, Jodi A., and Ariel A. Williamson. "Benefits of a Bedtime Routine in Young Children: Sleep, Development, and Beyond." *Sleep Medicine Reviews* 40 (2018): 93–108.

Newton, Adam T., Sarah M. Honaker, and Graham J. Reid. "Risk and Protective Factors and Processes for Behavioral Sleep Problems among Preschool and Early School-Aged Children: A Systematic Review." *Sleep Medicine Reviews* 52 (2020): 101303.

Nixon, Gillian M., John M. D. Thompson, Dug Yeo Han, David M. O. Becroft, Phillipa M. Clark, Elizabeth Robinson, Karen E. Waldie, Chris J. Wild, Peter N. Black, and Edwin A. Mitchell. "Falling Asleep: The Determinants of Sleep Latency." *Archives of Disease in Childhood* 94, no. 9 (2009): 686–89.

Nutt, David, Sue Wilson, and Louise Paterson. "Sleep Disorders as Core Symptoms of Depression." *Dialogues in Clinical Neuroscience* (2022).

Ong, Jason C., Rachel Manber, Zindel Segal, Yinglin Xia, Shauna Shapiro, and James K. Wyatt. "A Randomized Controlled Trial of Mindfulness Meditation for Chronic Insomnia." *Sleep* 37, no. 9 (2014): 1553–63.

Owens, Judith A., Anthony Spirito, Melissa McGuinn, and Chantelle Nobile. "Sleep Habits and Sleep Disturbance in Elementary School-Aged Children." *Journal of Developmental and Behavioral Pediatrics* 21, no. 1 (2000): 27–36.

Pandi-Perumal, Seithikurippu R., Jaime M. Monti, Deepa Burman, Ramanujam Karthikeyan, Ahmed S. BaHammam, David Warren Spence, Gregory M. Brown, and Meera Narashimhan. "Clarifying the Role of Sleep in Depression: A Narrative Review." *Psychiatry Research* 291 (2020): 113239.

Price, Anna M. H., Melissa Wake, Obioha C. Ukoumunne, and Harriet Hiscock. "Five-Year Follow-Up of Harms and Benefits of Behavioral Infant Sleep Intervention: Randomized Trial." *Pediatrics* 130, no. 4 (2012): 643–51.

Rapin, Lucile, Rihab Gamaoun, Cynthia El Hage, Maria Fernanda Arboleda, and Erin Prosk. "Cannabidiol Use and Effectiveness: Real-World Evidence from a Canadian Medical Cannabis Clinic." *Journal of Cannabis Research* 3, no. 1 (2021): 1–10.

Richter, David, Michael D. Krämer, Nicole K. Y. Tang, Hawley E. Montgomery-Downs, and Sakari Lemola. "Long-Term Effects of Pregnancy and Childbirth on Sleep Satisfaction and Duration of First-Time and Experienced Mothers and Fathers." *Sleep* 42, no. 4 (2019): zsz015.

Roberts, Robert E., Catherine R. Roberts, and Irene G. Chen. "Functioning of Adolescents with Symptoms of Disturbed Sleep." *Journal of Youth and Adolescence* 30, no. 1 (2001): 1–18.

Sack, Robert L., Dennis Auckley, R. Robert Auger, Mary A. Carskadon, Kenneth P. Wright Jr., Michael V. Vitiello, and Irina V. Zhdanova. "Circadian Rhythm Sleep Disorders: Part II, Advanced Sleep Phase Disorder, Delayed Sleep Phase Disorder, Free-Running Disorder, and Irregular Sleep-Wake Rhythm." *Sleep* 30, no. 11 (2007): 1484–501.

Sanvictores, Terrence, and Magda D. Mendez. "Types of Parenting Styles and Effects on Children" (2021). StatPearls. PMID: 33760502.

Schwartz, Daniel J., William C. Kohler, and Gillian Karatinos. "Symptoms of Depression in Individuals with Obstructive Sleep Apnea May Be Amenable to Treatment with Continuous Positive Airway Pressure." *Chest* 128, no. 3 (2005): 1304–9.

Scott, Alexander J., Thomas L. Webb, Marrissa Martyn-St James, Georgina Rowse, and Scott Weich. "Improving Sleep Quality Leads to Better Mental Health: A Meta-Analysis of Randomised Controlled Trials." *Sleep Medicine Reviews* 60 (2021): 101556.

Suni, Eric, and A. Singh. "How Much Sleep Do We Really Need." *Sleep Foundation* (2021).

Suraev, Anastasia S., Nathaniel S. Marshall, Ryan Vandrey, Danielle McCartney, Melissa J. Benson, Iain S. McGregor, Ronald R. Grunstein, and Camilla M. Hoyos. "Cannabinoid Therapies in the Management of Sleep Disorders: A Systematic Review of Preclinical and Clinical Studies." *Sleep Medicine Reviews* 53 (2020): 101339.

U.S. Department of Health and Human Services. *Physical Activity Guidelines for Americans*, 2nd ed. Washington, DC: U.S. Department of Health and Human Services, 2018.

Vandekerckhove, Marie, and Yu-lin Wang. "Emotion, Emotion Regulation and Sleep: An Intimate Relationship." *AIMS Neuroscience* 5, no. 1 (2018): 1.

Van Dongen, Hans P. A., Greg Maislin, Janet M. Mullington, and David F. Dinges. "The Cumulative Cost of Additional Wakefulness: Dose-Response Effects on Neurobehavioral Functions and Sleep Physiology from Chronic Sleep Restriction and Total Sleep Deprivation." *Sleep* 26, no. 2 (2003): 117–26.

Wang, Feifei, and Szilvia Boros. "The Effect of Physical Activity on Sleep Quality: A Systematic Review." *European Journal of Physiotherapy* 23, no. 1 (2021): 11–18.

Watson, Nathaniel F., Jennifer L. Martin, Merrill S. Wise, Kelly A. Carden, Douglas B. Kirsch, David A. Kristo, Raman K. Malhotra et al. "Delaying Middle School and High School Start Times Promotes Student Health and Performance: An American Academy of Sleep Medicine Position Statement." *Journal of Clinical Sleep Medicine* 13, no. 4 (2017): 623–25.

Weissbluth, Marc. *Healthy Sleep Habits, Happy Child: A Step-by-Step Program for a Good Night's Sleep*. New York: Ballantine Books, 2021.

Witbracht, Megan, Nancy L. Keim, Shavawn Forester, Adrianne Widaman, and Kevin Laugero. "Female Breakfast Skippers Display a Disrupted Cortisol Rhythm and Elevated Blood Pressure." *Physiology & Behavior* 140 (2015): 215–21.

Index

accommodations, 46; Anything Goes parenting and, 41–42; approaches to, 48, 49*t*–50*t*; safety behaviors, 132; term, 43

adaptability. *See* flexibility

adenoids, 16–17

adults. *See under* parent

alarms, bedwetting, 16

alcohol, and sleep, 165

American Academy of Child and Adolescent Psychiatry, 173

American Academy of Family Physicians, 173

American Academy of Pediatrics, 18, 173

American Academy of Sleep Medicine, 17, 173

American Psychological Association, 173

antihistamines, 22–23, 166; and alcohol, 165

anxiety: accommodation and, 42; in adults, 159; and bedtime issues, 148–49; transition steps for, 99–100

Anything Goes parenting, 41–43; and accommodations, 48, 49*t*–50*t*

apps: CBT-i Coach, 169; meditation, 168; sleep tracking, 164

aromatherapy, 24

attention, versus rewards, 146

attention-deficit hyperactivity disorder, and movement disorders, 16

auditory cues, for bedtime expectations, 76–77

Balanced parenting, 43–45, 129; and accommodations, 48, 49*t*–50*t*; achieving, 46–51

bath/shower, 19

battles: identifying, 84–88; picking, 75–97; tailored transition plans for, 101–28; types of, 7–8 bed: association with sleep, 21, 70–71, 161–62; term, 3

bedroom: phone in, 150; practice being alone in, 71; special touches for, 94

bedtime, attitudes toward, 63–67

bedtime routines, 9; for adults, 163; benefits of, 19; child development and, 27–28; communication and, 75–77; consistent, 19–20; definition of, 19; feedback on, 141; implementation of, 88–95, 99–138; maintenance of, 139–43; preparation for, 88–92, 94–95; putting all together, 128–34; selection of, 28–29, 30f; strategies for, 75–84; success with, 139–55; transition steps for, 99–100

Bed Warmer, 85–86; example of transition for, 111–12; transition plan for, 110–11

bedwetting, 15–16

behavioral insomnia, 12–13

behavioral interventions, 79–81; and behavioral insomnia, 13; shaping, 78–79

Benadryl. See antihistamines

blue light, 22, 165

body scan, 168

Bonus Week, 157–72

books, for bedtime, 90, 91t

breathing, mindful, 55–58; for adults, 168–69; maintenance of, 140–41

breathing disorders, sleep-related, 16–17

bribery, 45; versus reward system, 82

caffeine, 25; adults and, 165; transition plan and, 101

Calm, 168

cannabis/cannabidiol (CBD), 167

celebration, 142–43, 153–54

Centers for Disease Control and Prevention (CDC), 158, 173–74

certificate of achievement, 153–54

child development, 27–28; and emotions, 35–38; parenting style and, 39

circadian rhythm, 10, 22; and sleep disorders, 17

clocks, 162

cognitive-behavioral therapy for insomnia (CBTi), 169; resources for, 174

cognitive function, sleep deprivation and, 160

cognitive restructuring, 65

communication: and bedtime changes, 88–92; and child independent sleep, 75–77; and Demander, 113–14; and experience of independent sleep, 141–42; and nightmares, 151; scary talk from child, 145–46; and sleep, 69*t*; and sleepovers, 148; timing of, 133

concerning talk from child, 145–46

confidence: and anxiety, 148–49; building, 3, 42–43, 81, 127, 142

confusional arousal, 14

consequences, 76

consistency, 20, 139–40

co-parenting: and consistency, 139–40; issues in, 152–53; and parenting styles, 48; and transition plan, 100

coping skills, 36–37, 78; building, 55–74, 130; and nightmares, 151; and nighttime fears, 149; refusal of, 147; reminders of, 71–72; and sleep environment, 71

cortisol, 25

co-sleeping, 41, 153; loss of, 88, 90

COVID-19 pandemic, 7, 23, 56

crutches/props, issues with, 21, 24, 70, 124–25

crying, 28; worsening over time, 144–45

cuddling. *See* togetherness

culture, and parenting style, 38

Curtain Caller, 86–87; example of transition for, 121–22; in maintenance phase, 143–44; transition plan for, 118–21

delayed sleep phase syndrome, 17

Demander, 86; example of transition for, 116–18; transition plan for, 112–16

Department of Health and Human Services, 27

Department of Veterans Affairs, 169

depression, and sleep issues, 159

discomfort, child's, tolerating, 81

discouragement, 131

distress, 28; management of, 113–15; Ritualizer and, 123; transition steps for, 99–100; worsening over time, 144–45

doctor consultations, 12; for adults, 169–70; for Ritualizer, 87

doubt, 152

effort, praising, 140

emotions, 35–38; communication and, 92; management of, 113–16, 119; nighttime, 133, 149–50; purpose of, 37; sleep and, 158–59

endorphins, 27

enuresis, nocturnal, 15–16

environmental factors, 10, 20–21; for adults, 161–62; improving, 67–72; and sleep quality, 18

essential oils, 24

exercise: for adults, 163–64; and sleep, 27; timing of, 165

expectations, communication of, 75–77

extinction burst, 80–81, 95, 118; in maintenance phase, 144–45

fat, diets high in, and sleep, 25

fears: in adults, 159; child on, 90–92, 141–42; facing, 42; nighttime, tips for, 149–50

fight-or-flight system, 77–78

flexibility, 83–84; versus consistency, 139; Ritualizer and, 87–88, 123–24

Food and Drug Administration, 23

hangover effect, antihistamines and, 23

Headspace, 168

Host, 84–85; example of transition for, 104–5; transition plan for, 102–4

Ideal Bedtime Routine, 30*f,* 134–35

ignoring, planned, 79–81, 119

independent sleep: maintenance of, 139–43; strategies for, 75–84

interloper, dealing with, 143–44

light: and circadian rhythm, 22, 165; night-lights, 20, 78, 127–28; and sleep environment, 71, 161–62; transition plan and, 101

limit-setting insomnia, 12–13

magical solutions, 131–32

magnesium, 25

maintenance, 139–55

marijuana, 167

massage, 19

meaningful praise, 44, 93–94; and maintenance, 140

medications: and alcohol, 165; antihistamines, 22; caffeine in, 25; sleeping pills, 23–24. *See also* sleep aids

meditation, 162
melatonin, 22–23; for adults, 166; and alcohol, 165; nuts and, 24–25
Mental Health Foundation, 174
mental health issues, sleep deprivation and, 159
middle of night: adult awakenings, 162, 167–69; child visits, 107–8, 143–44
mindful breathing, 55–58; for adults, 168–69; maintenance of, 140–41
mindset, sleep-promoting, 63–67
mistakes, versus consistency, 144
mortality, sleep and, 160
movement disorders, sleep-related, 16
muscle relaxation, progressive, 58–63, 168
Musk, Elon, 158

naps: adults and, 166; and night sleep issues, 150
National Heart, Lung, and Blood Institute, 164, 170
National Sleep Foundation, 17, 18*t*, 174
nicotine, 165
night-lights, 20, 127–28; shaping and, 78

nightmare disorder, 15
nightmares, 150–51
night terrors, 14–15
nocturnal enuresis, 15–16
noise: building and, 92; and sleep environment, 67–70
No Nonsense parenting, 39–40
non-REM sleep, 11
nonverbal messaging, on sleep, 69*t*
nutrition: and sleep, 24–27, 26*t*; transition plan and, 101
nuts, and sleep, 24–25

Obama, Barack, 158
obsessive-compulsive disorder (OCD), 87
obstructive sleep apnea, 16–17
oversleeping, 169–70

parasomnias, 13–16
parent attitudes: doubt, 152; toward sleep, 66–67, 158, 160; toward togetherness, 151–52; toward transition plan, 101
parent behaviors, 9; responding to misbehavior, 113; tolerating child's discomfort, 81; what not to do, 131–34
parenting styles, 35–53; tracker for, 47*f*, 51–52; warmth and firmness in, 46*t*

parent sleep, 157–72; Curtain
Caller and, 120–21
periodic limb movement
disorder, 16
permissive parenting. *See*
Anything Goes parenting
perseverance, 133–34
phone, in bedroom, 150
Plan. *See* Transition Plan
planned ignoring, 79–81, 119
positive reinforcement,
44–45, 116
post-bedtime interactions: Bed
Warmer and, 111; Curtain
Caller and, 86–87, 118–21;
Host and, 103; limiting,
79; in maintenance phase,
143–44; Roommate and,
107–8
posters, inspirational, 72–73
praise, 44; and maintenance,
140; meaningful, 93–94; as
reward, 82
problem-solving, 90
Progressive Muscle Relaxation
(PMR), 58–63, 168
punishment, 45, 131

Quiet Check method, 119–20

rapid eye movement (REM)
sleep, 11, 159, 166
reassurance, 129–30; selectively
withholding, 81–82, 133

relaxation skills, 55–63; for
adults, 168; building, 130;
maintenance of, 140–41;
refusal of, 147
resources, 5, 170; for bedtime
books, 90, 91*t*; Bedtime
Routine worksheets, 31;
for CBTi, 174; certificate
of achievement, 153–54;
inspirational posters, 72–73;
Parenting Style worksheet,
51; Reward Chart, 96; for
sleep, 173–74; Transition
Plan worksheet, 100,
134–35
restless leg syndrome, 16
rewards, reward system,
82–83; Chart for, 96;
and Demander, 114;
development of, 93–94;
examples of, 95*t*; lack of
progress with, 146; and
nighttime roaming, 144
Ritualizer, 87–88; example
of transition for, 125–27;
transition plan for, 122–25
rituals: goodnight, 103–4; for
togetherness, 77
Roommate, 85; example of
transition for, 108–10;
transition plan for, 106–8
routines. *See* bedtime routines

safety behaviors, 132

scary talk from child, 145–46
school age, definition of, 36
school start times, 17–18
scripts: for introducing bedtime changes, 89; for mindful breathing, 57–58; for progressive muscle relaxation, 60–63; for saying goodnight, 79
self-regulation strategies, 77–78
separation anxiety, 148–49
serotonin, 168
shaping, 78–79, 119, 130–31
sleep, 7–33, 89, 134; benefits of, 170; positive messages on, 68*t*–69*t*; recommended amounts of, 17–18, 18*t*, 169–70; resources on, 173–74; script on, 89
sleep aids, 22–24; adults and, 166–67; and alcohol, 165; dependence on, 24, 70, 124–25; shaping and, 78–79; transition plan and, 101
sleep cycle, 11
sleep deprivation: costs of, 158–60; prevalence of, 158
sleep diary, 164, 170
sleep disorders, childhood, 12–17
Sleep Foundation, 174

sleeping pills, 167; contraindicated for children, 23–24
sleep issues: child, 1, 7; parent, 157–58; prevention of, 153
Sleep Junkies, 174
sleep onset association insomnia, 13, 21
sleepovers: bedwetting and, 15; sleep aids and, 24; tips for, 147–48
sleep quality, 18
sleep schedule, 161
sleep stories, 24
sleep terrors, 14–15
sleep tracking device, 164
sleep-wake homeostasis, 10
sleepwalking, 14
snacks, 24–27, 163; and sleep, 24–27, 26*t*; transition plan and, 101
Society of Behavioral Sleep Medicine, 174
Step-by-Step Transition Plan. *See* Transition Plan
strategies: for awakenings, 167–69; for independent sleep, 75–84; refusal of, 147; self-regulation, 77–78
stretching, 168
structure: definition of, 76; and independent sleep, 75–77
sugar, and sleep, 25

technology: and circadian rhythm, 22; and meditation, 168; phone in bedroom, 150; and sleep environment, 20, 71; sleep tracking device, 164; transition plan and, 100–101

temperature: for adults, 161; and sleep environment, 20, 67; transition plan and, 101

threatening talk from child, 145–46

title for child, 93

togetherness, 128–29, 132–33, 147, 151–52; Host and, 103; ritualizing, 77

tonsils, 16–17

Transition Plan: implementing, 88–95, 99–138; preparation for, 88–92, 94–95; putting all together, 128–34; start date for, 88, 100; tailored, 101–28; timing of, 100; worksheet for, 100, 134–35

troubleshooting, 143–53

Trump, Donald, 158

upsetting talk from child, 145–46

virtual assistive device, and bedtime cues, 76–77

visual cues, for bedtime expectations, 76–77

Week 1, 7–33

Week 2, 35–53

Week 3, 55–74

Week 4, 75–97

Week 5, 99–138

Week 6, 139–55

weighted blankets, 24

worksheets: Bedtime Routine, 31; Parenting Style, 51; Transition Plan, 100, 134–35

worry journal/time, 149–50; for adults, 162–63

You're On Your Own parenting, 40

About the Authors

Ellen Flannery-Schroeder, PhD, ABPP, is a licensed psychologist who specializes in anxiety disorders in children, efficacy of cognitive-behavioral treatment and prevention programs for children at risk for anxiety, parent training, and the role of family factors in anxiety disorders. Ellen earned her doctorate in clinical psychology at Temple University in 1997 and works as professor of psychology and director of the clinical psychology program at the University of Rhode Island. She has been involved in the prevention and treatment of anxiety disorders for more than thirty years and has written numerous articles and book chapters on the topic. Ellen directs the Child Anxiety Program in the Psychological Consultation Center at the University of Rhode Island; co-directs the New England Center for Anxiety, an outpatient treatment center in Rhode Island; co-directs High Performance Parenting, a parenting consultation firm; and helped to found The Greatest 8™ (thegreatest8.org), an initiative designed to promote mental health and wellness among children aged zero to eight. Additionally, Ellen conducts behavior change programming for former NFL players, is frequently invited to give paid talks and seminars, and has made numerous media appearances, including television, radio, newspaper, and podcast.

Chelsea Tucker, PhD, is a licensed psychologist with ten years of experience treating children and families seeking behavior change. She specializes in the cognitive-behavioral treatment of anxiety and anxiety-related issues in children, adolescents, and adults, with a focus on the role of family factors in the onset and maintenance of anxiety. Chelsea graduated with honors from the University of Rhode Island where she double-majored in psychology and Spanish language and literature. She earned her doctorate in school psychology at the University of Rhode Island in 2017. Chelsea currently practices at the New England Center for Anxiety, and she is founder and co-director of the CBT-based consultation firm, High Performance Parenting (highperformance-parenting.com).